In-Flight Medical Emergencies

Jose V. Nable • William Brady

Editors

In-Flight Medical Emergencies

A Practical Guide to Preparedness and Response

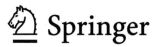 Springer

Editors
Jose V. Nable
Department of Emergency Medicine
MedStar Georgetown University Hospital
Georgetown University
Washington, DC
USA

William Brady
Department of Emergency Medicine
University of Virginia
Charlottesville, VA
USA

ISBN 978-3-319-74233-5   ISBN 978-3-319-74234-2   (eBook)
https://doi.org/10.1007/978-3-319-74234-2

Library of Congress Control Number: 2018934716

Printed on acid-free paper

This Springer imprint is published by the registered company Springer International Publishing AG part of Springer Nature
The registered company address is: Gewerbestrasse 11, 6330 Cham, Switzerland

Foreword

As a former Naval Flight Surgeon, trained in the US Navy, and having served in the French Naval Aviation, I faced many challenges with my patients worldwide in the air, at sea, in remote and hostile environments, in emergency departments, then later on expedition cruise ships and oil and gas operations. Making the right decision with limited information and resources in a complex environment summarizes in-flight medical practice. Earlier in my career, I would have indeed benefitted greatly in these environments from this Reference Book that Drs. Jose V. Nable and William Brady are offering to the medical community.

Having worked and traveled across the globe, I had my share of in-flight emergencies as a flight surgeon in Search and Rescue Missions, but also as a passenger responding to such events on commercial aircraft. On one occasion, in fact, I had to manage two significant medical emergencies in two connecting, consecutive flights. Indeed, in-flight emergencies do occur and more often than expected! As healthcare providers, we ethically and dutifully assist as critical first responders in these situations. To implement a best practice standard in this unique environment, one needs to be prepared. In a plane cruising at 36,000 ft, with the nearest medical facility sometimes hours away, if any, and with weather and flight limitations, rapid ad hoc medical management is critical for the patient but also for the multiple passengers who are sharing a confined cabin. Then there are the related international legal and liability issues to remember! This book is a survival kit for all physicians and other healthcare providers, whatever their specialty, because as we board the plane as a passenger, we ethically have to respond to assist in medical emergencies.

Onboard a commercial aircraft, like on a ship, we have to remember that the captain is ultimately responsible to make the final decision impacting the health and welfare of his or her passengers. We can only offer our best medical advice and technical support for the patient, relying on our own personal skill limitations and scant medical tools available. This realization is significant for the physician and many other healthcare providers, recognizing that medical decisions are not ultimately ours.

I am now working daily on arranging air repatriations (i.e., nonurgent commercial air travel) for our patients worldwide with Dr. Brady and his esteemed colleagues. Technical, legal, fiscal, logistical, and security issues can make the simplest medical case a massive challenge! In this book, the editors have assembled a knowledgeable and experienced cadre of authors who share a unique "know-how," which will provide the reader recommendations, evidence-based when possible. The contents of the book address the necessary topics to be comfortable to understand the specificity of these in-flight medical situations. If you need just one user guide for in-flight medical emergencies, this is the one.

Beyond the individual use of this book, the extensive range of the topics covered provides physicians, other healthcare providers, and hospital administrators the knowledge to better understand the unique challenges in these patient movements by air; institutions and groups who are facing medical challenges in their area of operations (government and nongovernment organizations, cruise lines, oil and gas companies, expatriates, etc…) will be able to better assess the medical risks and necessary mitigation measures when integrating the latest update of in-flight care. Passengers-to-be with the range of medical conditions, who have questions about their ability to fly, will also benefit when their primary care physician consults this text.

We, as medical providers and commercial aircraft passengers, are at the forefront of this air medical frontier. This frontier is changing rapidly due to the growth in commercial aviation, the wider use of aircrafts as medical vectors, and the upgrade of medical tools available onboard and related level of care that can be achieved today when sitting 36,000 feet above ground.

I highly recommend using this book as your guide when traveling because it is not a matter of "if" you will need it, but "when" you will need it!

Bruno Sicard, M.D., Ph.D.
Chief Medical Officer
Allianz Global Assistance Canada
Allianz Medical Global Competence Center
Americas Zone
Kitchener, ON
Canada

Preface

Picture yourself on a flight from New York to Los Angeles. The plane is at cruising altitude. You just started to watch a movie you had been looking forward to on your handheld device. Even though you're wearing headphones, your attention is drawn away from the movie when you hear several tones on the overhead speaker followed by the announcement. "Attention all passengers, if there is a medical doctor on board, please ring your call button. Once again, if there is a medical doctor on board, please ring your call button."

Thoughts race through your head. Should I volunteer? Should I wait to see if other volunteers come forward? What sort of medical kit is on the plane? What medical training do the flight attendants have? What if this person is critically ill? What if it involves a child? You quickly run through a list of potential medical emergencies that could await you, but you take a deep breath and press your call button anyway. You have now entered the world of providing medical assistance to patients suffering in an in-flight emergency.

Providing medical assistance during a flight offers a number of unique challenges including lower cabin pressure, tight quarters, crowded conditions, and loud background noise. The purpose of this text is to offer an overview of the sort of in-flight emergencies that could be anticipated and to outline treatment priorities, should you be the one who presses their call button to volunteer. The book describes the physical environment inside the cabin, some medicolegal issues, problems unique to international flights, the various medical conditions that are common, as well as measures that can be taken by passengers with medical conditions in preparation for flight. The book also contains sections on ground-based medical direction of in-flight emergencies and the use of commercial aircraft for medical evacuations.

While in-flight medical emergencies are relatively rare with the rate of occurrence of one in 11,000 passengers, the sheer number of passengers makes it very likely that you will one day be summoned to render assistance. This is especially true if you travel with any regularity. This book is a must-read for the medical professional who would contemplate volunteering to render medical assistance during a flight and offers an excellent introduction to medical care in the austere and remote environment of the aircraft cabin.

After reading this book, you are able to deliver the needed medical assistance thus preempting emergency measures. The flight attendants are thankful; the other passengers are in awe; you are able to return to your seat. Now back to that movie.

Charlottesville, VA, USA   Robert E. O'Connor, M.D., M.P.H.

Contents

About the Editors

Jose V. Nable, M.D., M.S., NRP   is Assistant Professor of Emergency Medicine at Georgetown University School of Medicine and MedStar Georgetown University Hospital. He is Medical Director at Georgetown Emergency Response Medical Service. He is a nationally registered paramedic with significant experience in delivering medical care in the out-of-hospital setting.

William Brady, M.D.   is Professor of Emergency Medicine and Internal Medicine at the University of Virginia School of Medicine and the David A. Harrison Distinguished Educator. He is the Medical Director of Emergency Management of the UVA Health System and Operational Medical Director of Albemarle County Fire Rescue. He has worked extensively in travel medicine and related in-flight medical events.

Contributors

B. Barrie Bostick, M.D. Department of Emergency Medicine, University of Maryland Upper Chesapeake Medical Center, Bel Air, MD, USA

Matthew Beardmore, M.B., Ch.B. (Hons) Department of Anesthesiology, Peninsula Deanery, Plymouth, UK

Lisa Bowman, R.N., B.S.N., C.E.N. Emergency Department, University of Virginia Medical Center, Charlottesville, VA, USA

William Brady, M.D. Department of Emergency Medicine, University of Virginia, Charlottesville, VA, USA

Lauren B. Brady, B.S.Ed., M.S.Ed. School of Medicine, University of Virginia, Charlottesville, VA, USA

Wan-Tsu W. Chang, M.D. Department of Emergency Medicine, University of Maryland School of Medicine, Baltimore, MD, USA

Christin Child, R.N., B.S.N., C.E.N. Emergency Department, University of Virginia Medical Center, Charlottesville, VA, USA

Thomas J. Doyle, M.D., M.P.H. Department of Emergency Medicine, University of Pittsburgh School of Medicine, Pittsburgh, PA, USA

Sarah B. Dubbs, M.D. Department of Emergency Medicine, University of Maryland School of Medicine, Baltimore, MD, USA

University of Maryland Medical Center, Baltimore, MD, USA

François-Xavier Duchateau, M.D. Allianz Worldwide Partners, Group Medical Direction, Saint Ouen, France

Jason M. Franasiak, M.D., FACOG, HCLD/ALD (ABB) Reproductive Medicine Associates of New Jersey, Sidney Kimmel Medical College—Thomas Jefferson University, Philadelphia, PA, USA

Tobias Gauss, M.D. HEMS, East Anglian Air Ambulance, Norwich, UK

John Gilday, R.N., M.S.N., NREMT-P Department of Emergency Services, University of Virginia Medical Center, Charlottesville, VA, USA

J. Gregory Webb, Esq. MichieHamlett PLLC (Attorneys at Law), Charlottesville, VA, USA

Sara A. Hefton, M.D. Department of Neurological Surgery, Division of Neuro-Trauma and Critical Care, Thomas Jefferson University, Philadelphia, PA, USA

Kami M. Hu, M.D. Departments of Emergency Medicine and Internal Medicine, University of Maryland School of Medicine, Baltimore, MD, USA

Priya Kuppusamy, M.D. Department of Emergency Medicine, University of Maryland School of Medicine, Baltimore, MD, USA

E. Kyle McNew, Esq. MichieHamlett PLLC (Attorneys at Law), Charlottesville, VA, USA

Christian Martin-Gill, M.D., M.P.H. Department of Emergency Medicine, University of Pittsburgh School of Medicine, Pittsburgh, PA, USA

Edward Meyers, R.N., B.S., M.S.N., EMT-I Department of Emergency Services, University of Virginia Medical Center, Charlottesville, VA, USA

Terrence Mulligan, D.O., M.P.H. Department of Emergency Medicine, University of Maryland School of Medicine, Baltimore, MD, USA

Jose V. Nable, M.D., M.S., NRP Department of Emergency Medicine, MedStar Georgetown University Hospital, Georgetown University, Washington, DC, USA

Tu Carol Nguyen, D.O. Emergency Department, University of Maryland Prince George's Hospital Center, Cheverly, MD, USA

Robert E. O'Connor, M.D., M.P.H. University of Virginia School of Medicine, Charlottesville, VA, USA

Geoffrey A. Ramin, M.B.B.S., F.A.C.E.M. Allianz Worldwide Partners, Brisbane, QLD, Australia

Sarah K. Sommerkamp, M.D., R.D.M.S. University of Maryland Midtown Campus, Baltimore, MD, USA

Department of Emergency Medicine, University of Maryland School of Medicine, Baltimore, MD, USA

Ryan Spangler, M.D. Department of Emergency Medicine, University of Maryland School of Medicine, Baltimore, MD, USA

Kathleen Stephanos, M.D. Department of Emergency Medicine, Strong Memorial Hospital, Rochester, NY, USA

Sara F. Sutherland, M.D., M.B.A. University of Virginia School of Medicine, Charlottesville, VA, USA

Christina L. Tupe, M.D. Emergency Medicine, Prince George's Hospital Center, Cheverly, MD, USA

Emergency Medicine, University of Maryland Upper Chesapeake Medical Center, Bel Air, MD, USA

Laurent Verner, M.D. Allianz Worldwide Partners, Group Medical Direction, Saint Ouen, France

Setting the Scene

1

Jose V. Nable and William Brady

1.1 Introduction

"One of our passengers is experiencing a medical emergency. Is there a doctor on-board? If so, please press your flight attendant call button." For a healthcare provider who travels on a commercial airliner, hearing this query may instill a bit of trepidation. Many questions may come to mind:

- What is my role as a volunteering healthcare provider?
- What resources are available to me?
- What liability issues surround responding?
- Am I required to respond?
- What types of emergencies might I expect to encounter?

Medical professionals are not uncommonly called upon to use their skills in the non-clinical environment. Flying in an aircraft, however, may present unique challenges. As one is flying in a cramped metal tube at an altitude of 35,000 ft, medical care is truly a form of austere medicine. In this book, we will attempt to answer many of these previously posed questions. We hope that readers will be able to confidently handle medical issues that may arise during a flight. We also will discuss how healthcare providers may potentially prevent or mitigate the development of acute medical events in their patients who are about to embark on a journey.

J. V. Nable, M.D., M.S., NRP (✉)
Department of Emergency Medicine, MedStar Georgetown University Hospital,
Georgetown University, Washington, DC, USA
e-mail: Jose.Nable@georgetown.edu

W. Brady, M.D.
Department of Emergency Medicine, University of Virginia, Charlottesville, VA, USA
e-mail:wb4z@virginia.edu

© Springer International Publishing AG, part of Springer Nature 2018
J. V. Nable, W. Brady (eds.), *In-Flight Medical Emergencies*,
https://doi.org/10.1007/978-3-319-74234-2_1

1.2   History of Handling In-Flight Medical Events

In 1930, Boeing Air Transport, predecessor to today's United Airlines, flew the first commercial flight in the United States with a female flight attendant [1]. The pioneering flight attendant, Ellen Church, was both a pilot and a nurse. Church had encouraged the airline to hire nurses as flight attendants, with the hope that their nursing skills and rapport could provide a sense of security to passengers, who were somewhat fearful of flight during the airline industry's early days [2]. Church set a precedent; before World War II, nearly all American flight attendants were nurses [3–5].

In those early days of commercial airline travel, these onboard nurses also somewhat served a second function: their ability to assist with an unexpected in-flight medical event. Indeed, newspapers not uncommonly reported contemporaneous reports of passengers experiencing medical emergencies during flight [6, 7].

By World War II, however, the general rule that flight attendants be nurses was dropped to divert their efforts to the war [8]. Thereafter, flight crews commonly asked for volunteer healthcare providers to assist with passengers experiencing a medical event [9]. Providers, however, were often volunteering without clear knowledge of their liability and minimal onboard medical resources [9].

Until the 1980s, onboard medical equipment typically only included bandages, aspirin, acetaminophen, and an antihistamine [10]. As such, the American Medical Association historically suggested that physicians who travel may carry an improvised medical kit that included diagnostic equipment (such as a blood pressure cuff) and a cache of injectable medications such as epinephrine, atropine, and diazepam [10]. The US Federal Aviation Administration (FAA) in 1986 finally mandated that airlines carry an expanded cache of medical supplies, including injectable dextrose, epinephrine, nitroglycerin tablets, syringes, needles, and oropharyngeal airways [11]. Before this expansion of onboard emergency medical kits, many airlines operated under the premise that an expedited landing was the best course of action for passengers experiencing an acute medical issue [12].

This somewhat-expanded medical kit was, however, still notably minimal. The increasing availability of automated external defibrillators (AEDs), in particular, suggested that the FAA's mandated kit of 1986 could be further expanded [13]. In 1998, the US Congress passed the Aviation Medical Assistance Act (AMAA). This act required the FAA to reevaluate the mandatory contents of onboard medical supplies [14]. In response to the AMAA, the FAA further expanded the kit in 2001 to contain the supplies listed in Table 1.1. In addition, US airlines were also required to carry AEDs [15].

The AMAA also provided responding providers with liability protection [14]. The act was meant to encourage traveling healthcare professionals to respond to in-flight medical events by standardizing medical equipment aboard aircraft and shielding providers from potential legal liability.

Table 1.1 Contents of Emergency Medical Kits Required by the Federal Aviation Administration to be Present on All Commercial Airliners Based in the United States [15]

Contents	Quantity
Sphygmomanometer	1
Stethoscope	1
Airways, oropharyngeal (3 sizes): 1 pediatric, 1 small adult, 1 large adult, or equivalent	3
Self-inflating manual resuscitation device with 3 masks (1 pediatric, 1 small adult, 1 large adult, or equivalent)	3
CPR mask (3 sizes), 1 pediatric, 1 small adult, 1 large adult, or equivalent	3
IV Admin Set: Tubing w/2 Y connectors	1
Alcohol sponges	2
Adhesive tape, 1-in. standard roll adhesive	1
Tape scissors	1
Tourniquet	1
Saline solution, 500 cm^3	1
Protective nonpermeable gloves or equivalent	1
Needles (2–18 gauge, 2–20 gauge, 2–22 gauge, or sizes necessary to administer required medications)	6
Syringes (1–5 cm^3, 2–10 cm^3, or sizes necessary to administer required medications)	4
Analgesic, nonnarcotic, tablets, 325 mg	4
Antihistamine tablets, 25 mg	4
Antihistamine injectable, 50 mg (single-dose ampule or equivalent)	2
Atropine, 0.5 mg, 5 cm^3 (single-dose ampule or equivalent)	2
Aspirin tablets, 325 mg	4
Bronchodilator, inhaled (metered-dose inhaler or equivalent)	1
Dextrose, 50%/50 cm^3 injectable (single-dose ampule or equivalent)	1
Epinephrine 1:1,000, 1 cm^3, injectable (single-dose ampule or equivalent)	2
Epinephrine 1:10,000, 2 cm^3, injectable (single-dose ampule or equivalent)	2
Lidocaine, 5 cm^3, 20 mg/mL, injectable (single-dose ampule or equivalent)	2
Nitroglycerine tablets, 0.4 mg	10
Basic instructions for use of the drugs in the kit	1

1.3 Epidemiology of In-Flight Medical Events

As there is no mandatory centralized reporting system for in-flight medical events, it is difficult to estimate the frequency of these occurrences [16]. Before the FAA adopted its most recent final ruling on the contents of onboard emergency medical kits, some industry stakeholders suggested the adoption of a tracking system for all events be implemented [15]. The FAA did not adopt this suggestion, noting that the collection of comprehensive data could overburden airline carriers without any clear benefit. As long-term outcome data of a treated passenger would be inaccessible to airlines and the government, the FAA contended that a reporting system would likely yield little information. While the adoption of a reporting system has also been suggested by researchers [16], the Aerospace Medical Association has noted that such a system would likely be costly and logistically challenging to implement [17].

Some data on in-flight medical events, however, can be gleaned from the literature. Researchers, for example, queried the database of a ground-based medical consultation service that provides flight crews with real-time guidance for handling onboard medical events. In this study, the most common incidents included syncope (accounting for 37.4% of consultations), respiratory issues (12.1%), nausea or vomiting (9.5%), cardiac issues (77%), seizures (5.8%), and abdominal pain (4.1%) [18]. The same study estimated that medical events reported to the consultation service occur in 1 out of every 604 flights [18]. It should be noted, however, that a reporting bias likely exists. Many in-flight medical events are potentially handled by flight crews and onboard healthcare providers without ever consulting resources on the ground.

Deaths of passengers who have an in-flight medical emergency are exceedingly rare, with the Aerospace Medical Association estimating a mortality rate of 0.1 deaths per million passengers, or approximately 0.3% of in-flight medical emergencies [19]. A true estimate, however, is difficult to ascertain, as the underlying studies behind this estimate were challenged to account for deaths that occurred after transfer of patients to definitive care [18, 20].

1.4   Onboard Medical Resources

In the event of an in-flight medical emergency, responding healthcare providers can and should request that the flight crew make available the onboard emergency medical kit and AED (if appropriate). While the contents of the expanded medical kit were previously discussed in Table 1.1, other basic supplies are generally also available, such as bandages and splints to care for minor trauma.

The resources of the emergency medical kit are certainly not all-encompassing. For example, there are no drugs suitable for handling acute psychiatric issues, despite such events constituting an estimated 3.5% of in-flight medical emergencies [21]. There are also no pediatric-appropriate supplies [22]. Obstetric supplies are notably absent as well.

Healthcare providers who respond to onboard events are indeed practicing austere medicine. Providers may need to improvise or solicit supplies from other passengers. For example, if a passenger is suspected of being hypoglycemic, a responding provider might find it suitable to request for a glucometer from other passengers, keeping in mind that true calibration and ensuring of cleanliness of such borrowed devices may be impossible.

Because of the somewhat limited medical supplies aboard commercial aircraft, professional societies and other interested parties have petitioned the government to further expand the medical cache. The Aerospace Medical Association, for example, has endorsed a guidance document recommending that airlines carry antipsychotics, antiepileptics, diuretics, and steroids [17]. In 2015, a bill was introduced in the US Congress to mandate that airlines carry epinephrine auto-injectors [23].

The FAA has indicated, however, that the emergency medical kits are not meant to supply a flying medical clinic [15]. The federal government does not anticipate nor expect airlines to carry supplies for every single type of potential medical event. And while the mandated kit attempts to address the needs of several types of medical emergencies, not every type of emergency can reasonably be covered.

1.5 Ground-Based Consultation Services

Because healthcare providers are not necessarily available to assist on every flight, the vast majority of airlines contract with a ground-based medical consultation service [24]. These services are staffed by health professionals who provide guidance to flight crews on handling cases in real time. For example, if a passenger develops chest pain, flight attendants can contact providers on the ground to determine an appropriate plan, such as potential diversion of the flight.

Responding healthcare providers onboard the aircraft can likewise discuss acute medical events with these ground-based consultation services. If an onboard provider is uncertain about how to best handle a situation, that provider can consider conferring with the airline's contracted ground-based consultation service [25].

1.6 Challenges of In-Flight Medical Care

It is important for responding clinicians to understand the challenges associated with providing care in a commercial airline environment. Modern airlines provide passengers with increasingly cramped cabins. This leaves little room for a healthcare provider to adequately assess a passenger with an acute medical event. Unless the passenger is in first or business class, it may be impossible to recline the passenger without moving the patient to the floor, which may be necessary when treating a patient with shock physiology. Additionally, the confined condition of a modern airliner means that patient privacy cannot truly be ensured. Responding providers should make a concerted effort to respect a patient's privacy, such as using galleys or other areas of the aircraft not in the immediate vicinity of other passengers to perform potentially uncomfortable histories and physical exams.

In addition to cramped cabins, passengers are often already stressed by a prolonged check-in process and increasingly onerous security measures at the airport [26]. These stressful conditions can exacerbate underlying psychiatric issues or lead to "air rage" [27]. If a responding physician assesses the need for flight diversion, that provider should be prepared to be challenged by other passengers who understandably may be dismayed by the change in flight plans.

Another challenge of in-flight medical care is the previously mentioned lack of comprehensive medical supplies. Responding providers must be prepared to improvise to manage situations that are often easily handled in a clinical environment. As an example, a physician documented a case report of using a urinary catheter to perform a thoracostomy for patient experiencing a pneumothorax on a transcontinental flight [28]. The austere environment may challenge healthcare providers who are accustomed to working with easy access to medical supplies.

When flying on an international airline, the onboard medical kits will likely not conform to the standards to which US-based airlines must adhere. Drug names may be different. Acetaminophen, for instance, may be labeled as paracetamol. Liability issues are also potentially complicated when treating citizens of other countries on an airline not registered in the United States [24]. Also, unlike in the United States, several countries in Europe mandate that physicians respond to an acute onboard medical event [29].

Responding healthcare providers should also be mindful that they do not have supervisory authority over the flight crew when handling medical emergencies. According to the Montreal Convention and FAA regulations, the flight crew is ultimately responsible for activities aboard the aircraft [24, 30]. The crew may disagree with recommendations by onboard providers, choosing to accept conflicting advice from the airline's contracted ground-based consultation service. The crew also has discretion when allowing access to the emergency medical kit. The FAA does note that it would be "preferable" for airline personnel to check the credentials of volunteer responders who identify themselves as healthcare providers [30].

1.7   Diversion

Some passengers may experience an acute medical event in which flight diversion may be appropriate. Diversion potentially gives such passengers timelier access to critical definitive care. It is no surprise, then, that the most common medical complaints associated with diversion are related to cardiac, respiratory, and neurologic emergencies [18]. Issues involving these organ systems may have time-dependent treatments. For example, a passenger with sudden-onset hemiplegia may be experiencing a stroke, in which case timely administration of thrombolytics may improve that patient's neurologic outcome [31]. Or a passenger with chest pain and diaphoresis may be experiencing an ST-segment elevation myocardial infarction, wherein rapid access to a cardiac catheterization lab is essential [32].

Unfortunately, it is not possible to diagnose many of these time-sensitive conditions in the setting of the airline cabin environment. Responding onboard healthcare providers must therefore use clinical judgment, incorporating history, risk factors, and physical exam, to assess passengers experiencing high-risk complaints. If a clinician has a high index of suspicion for a condition in which rapid access to formal ground-based medical care is necessary, diversion of the aircraft may be appropriate.

Diverting an aircraft from its intended destination has significant consequences. In addition to being expensive (with one source estimating costs up to $500,000 to divert a large, fully-loaded aircraft [33]), diversion may force the airline to reroute the other passengers. Some aircraft may also need to dump excess fuel prior to an expedited landing [34]. Irrespective of these potential secondary effects, it is the professional responsibility of a clinician who assesses the need for quicker access to ground-based medical care to communicate that assessment with the flight crew.

Because of the complicated decision making surrounding diversion, many airlines will discuss a recommendation for an expedited landing with their contracted ground-based consultation service. The final decision for diversion ultimately rests with the captain of the aircraft [16].

1.8   Our Flight Path

This book will provide the reader with an understanding of various topics surrounding in-flight medical emergencies. The pathophysiology of flight is first discussed. Although thousands of flights occur daily in the United States, flight is not necessarily benign, particularly for those with preexisting medical conditions. The medicolegal issues that can occur when volunteering medical assistance will also be examined.

Several chapters are devoted to the various types of acute medical events that may occur during a flight. Recognizing when medical issues are potentially lethal, and in need of more rapid access to definitive medical care, is therein emphasized. For such conditions, the reader will be familiarized with temporizing treatments that may be available on board aircraft.

Finally, the book discusses treatments that may be available prior to flight to mitigate potential in-flight medical events. Additionally, the topic of medical clearance of passengers is presented.

References

1. Latson J. Hired for their looks, promoted for their heroism: the first flight attendants. In: Time magazine. 2015. http://time.com/3847732/first-stewardess-ellen-church/. Accessed 14 Nov 2016.
2. A 3-month airline experiment turns 50 years old: 13 stops in 20-hour flight. The New York Times; 1980 May 30: B16.
3. Gazdik M. Vault guide to flight attendant careers. New York: Vault; 2004.
4. Lockridge P. The transatlantic girls. The Washington Post; 1943 July 25: S10.
5. Ford E. Flying girls a vital part of air epic: airline stewardesses on D.C. runs are all former nurses. Duties on board plane are exciting and varied. The Washington Post; 1937 July 4: B4.
6. Stricken in plane, woman of 70 dies. The New York Times; 1945 Sept 14: 17.
7. Another baby born in plane over atlantic. The Washington Post; 1949 Nov 23: B10.
8. Tim K. The Flight Attendant Career Guide. River Forest, IL: Planning/Communications Publishing; 1995.
9. Yenckel JT. Is there a doctor in the plane? The Washington Post; 1995 July 9: E1.
10. American Medical Association Commission on Emergency Medical Services. Medical aspects of transportation aboard commercial aircraft. AMA commission on emergency medical services. JAMA. 1982;247(7):1007–11.
11. Department of transportation, federal aviation administration: emergency medical equipment requirement. Fed Regist. 1986;51:1218–1223.
12. McLellan D. Airlines gear up for medical emergencies. In: Los Angeles Times. 1986. http://articles.latimes.com/1986-06-05/news/vw-9535_1_medical-emergencies/3. Accessed 16 Nov 2016.
13. Nichol G, Hallstrom AP, Kerber R, et al. American Heart Association report on the second public access defibrillation conference, April 17-19, 1997. Circulation. 1998;97(13):1309–14.

14. Aviation Medical Assistance Act of 1998, Pub L. No. 105–170. Washington, DC: National Archives and Records Administration, 1998.
15. United States Federal Aviation Administration. Emergency medical equipment. Final rule. Fed Regist. 2001;66:19028–46.
16. Goodwin T. In-flight medical emergencies: an overview. BMJ. 2000;321:1338–41.
17. Aerospace Medical Association. Medical emergencies: managing in-flight medical events. 2016. https://www.asma.org/publications/medical-publications-for-airline-travel/managing-in-flight-medical-events. Accessed 1 Dec 2016.
18. Peterson DC, Martin-Gill C, Guyette FX, et al. Outcomes of medical emergencies on commercial airline flights. N Engl J Med. 2013;368:2075–83.
19. Thibeault C, Evans AD. Medical guidelines for air travel: reported in-flight medical events and death. Aerosp Med Hum Perform. 2015;86(6):571.
20. Delaune EF, Lucas RH, Illig P. In-fl ight medical events and aircraft diversions: one airline's experience. Aviat Space Environ Med. 2003;74(1):62–8.
21. Matsumoto K, Goebert D. In-flight psychiatric emergencies. Aviat Space Environ Med. 2001;72:919–23.
22. Moore BR, Ping JM, Claypool DW. Pediatric emergencies on a US-based commercial airline. Pediatr Emerg Care. 2005;21:725–9.
23. Airline access to emergency epinephrine act of 2015, S. 1972, 114th Cong. 2015.
24. Gendreau MA, DeJohn C. Responding to medical events during commercial airline flights. N Engl J Med. 2002;346:1067–73.
25. Rayman RB, Zanick D, Korsgard T. Resources for inflight medical care. Aviat Space Environ Med. 2004;75(3):278–80.
26. DeHart RL. Health issues of air travel. Annu Rev Public Health. 2003;24:133–51.
27. DeCelles KA, Norton MI. Physical and situational inequality on airplanes predicts air rage. Proc Natl Acad Sci U S A. 2016;113(20):5588–91.
28. Wallace TW, Wong T, O'Bichere A, Ellis BW. Managing in flight emergencies. BMJ. 1995;311(7001):374–6.
29. Kuczkowski KM. "Code blue" in the air: implications of rendering care during in-flight medical emergencies. Can J Anaesth. 2007;54(5):401–2.
30. United States Federal Aviation Administration. Advisory circular: emergency medical equipment. AC No. 121-33B; 2006.
31. National Institute of Neurological Disorders and Stroke rt-PA Stroke Study Group. Tissue plasminogen activator for acute ischemic stroke. N Engl J Med. 1995;333(24):1581–7.
32. Levine GN, Bates ER, Blankenship JC, et al. 2015 ACC/AHA/SCAI focused update on primary percutaneous coronary intervention for patients with ST-Elevation myocardial infarction: an update of the 2011 ACCF/AHA/SCAI guideline for percutaneous coronary intervention and the 2013 ACCF/AHA guideline for the management of ST-Elevation myocardial infarction. J Am Coll Cardiol. 2016;67(10):1235–50.
33. Bukowski JH, Richards JR. Commercial airline in-flight emergency: medical student response and review of medicolegal issues. J Emerg Med. 2016;50(1):74–8.
34. Hung KK, Cocks RA, Poon WK, et al. Medical volunteers in commercial flight medical diversions. Aviat Space Environ Med. 2013;84(5):491–7.

Pathophysiology of Flight

2

Geoffrey A. Ramin

2.1 Introduction

Humans were never intended to fly but the evolution of the aviation industry has meant that we can now easily overcome this limitation and, by utilising aircraft, be rapidly placed into a high-altitude environment. However, even within the protective shell of modern aircraft we will be exposed to a number of physiological changes. The human body has a remarkable capacity to compensate for these changes but their impact becomes increasingly significant when transporting sick or injured patients by air. The first step in understanding the implications of flight is to review the physics of the atmosphere and the behaviour of gases.

2.2 The Atmosphere

The atmosphere is made up of a mixture of gases, the bulk of which is comprised of nitrogen (78%) and oxygen (21%). The remaining 1% is made up of predominantly inert gases and a trace of carbon dioxide. Convective mixing of gases ensures that this percentage composition remains the same to over 10 km above sea level (ASL). This means that within this range of altitude, the fraction of inspired oxygen (FiO_2) will always be 21% or 0.21. This atmosphere also exerts weight as a result of the gravitational pull of the Earth. Whilst this can vary slightly with atmospheric conditions, standard atmospheric pressure at sea level is assumed to be 760 mmHg or 14.7 psi. Atmospheric pressure decreases with altitude, so whilst the FiO_2 remains constant with increasing altitude, the partial pressure exerted by oxygen in the atmosphere decreases.

G. A. Ramin, M.B.B.S., F.A.C.E.M.
Allianz Worldwide Partners, Brisbane, QLD, Australia
e-mail: ketamine@internode.on.net

Table 2.1 Physiological zones of the atmosphere

Zone	Altitude ASL (ft)	Atmospheric pressure (mmHg)	Features
Physiological	0–10,000	760–523	Ability for humans to compensate and maintain physiological efficiency
Deficient	10,000–50,000	523–87	Progressive hypoxia leading to failure of physiological compensation
Space Equivalent	>50,000	87–0	Environment hostile to humans and unable to maintain life

Whilst the atmosphere has physically distinct zones, all aeromedical operations would occur well within the troposphere, which extends to as low as 23,000 ft ASL at the poles and up to 65,000 ft ASL at the equator [1]. Of greater relevance medically, the atmosphere can also be divided into three physiological zones according to the effect of each on the body's physiological responses as shown in Table 2.1 [2, 3]. Aeromedical operations would generally occur well within the physiological zone where a fit and healthy individual maintains the ability to compensate and ensure physiologic efficiency with only minimal impairment seen in arterial oxygen transport. In this case, the changes in pressure on ascent and descent would only potentially cause minor discomfort in gas-containing regions such as the middle ear and sinuses. However, neither is necessarily the case for sick or injured patients where increasing altitude can lead to increased physiological compromise.

2.3 The Gas Laws

The molecules of any gas are in constant random motion and the pressure exerted by a gas or mixture of gases depends on the number of molecules, their velocity, and mass. As we ascend to higher altitude, the weight of the atmosphere above us decreases and there is an associated decrease in atmospheric pressure. As air is compressible, the pressure decreases more rapidly the higher we ascend. There are three principal gas laws that need to be reviewed in order to understand the implications of altitude on the human body in regard to the transport of sick or injured patients. These are Dalton's law, Boyle's law, and Henry's law [3, 4].

2.3.1 Dalton's Law

Also known as the law of partial pressures, Dalton's law states that in any mixture of gases, each individual gas will exert a pressure that is proportional to its concentration within that mixture and that the total pressure exerted by the mixture is the sum of each of these respective partial pressures. This can be expressed as

$P_t = P_1 + P_2 + \ldots\ldots\ldots P_n$

where P_t = Total pressure

P_1 to P_n = Partial pressure of each gas within the mixture

n = Total number of gases in the mixture

Table 2.2 Gas expansion ratios at varying altitude

Altitude ASL (ft)	Gas expansion ratio
Sea level	1.0
5,000	1.2
8,000	1.3
10,000	1.5
30,000	4.0
40,000	7.6

As you will recall, the standard pressure of the atmosphere at sea level is 760 mmHg, also referred to as 1 atmosphere. Oxygen comprises 21% of the atmospheric gas mixture. This percentage is referred to as the FiO_2 and, as per Dalton's law, the partial pressure of inspired oxygen (PiO_2) would therefore be 21% of 760 mmHg which equates to 160 mmHg. As altitude increases and atmospheric pressure falls so does the PiO_2. At 10,000 ft ASL, atmospheric pressure is only 523 mmHg resulting in a PiO_2 of 21% of 523 mmHg which equates to 110 mmHg. So, whilst as previously stated the FiO_2 remains constant with increasing altitude, the PiO_2 decreases significantly.

2.3.2 Boyle's Law

Boyle's law states that, at a constant temperature, the volume of a gas will vary inversely with pressure. Therefore, as atmospheric pressure decreases, there is an increase in gas volume. This can be expressed as

$P_1 \times V_1 = P_2 \times V_2$

where P_1 = initial pressure, V_1 = initial volume

P_2 = new pressure, V_2 = new volume

Utilising Boyle's law, we can calculate that the volume of a gas in an enclosed space at sea level would expand to ~1.5 times its original volume at 10,000 ft ASL. Table 2.2 shows the typical gas expansion ratios at varying altitudes.

2.3.3 Henry's Law

Henry's law states that, at a constant temperature, the volume of a gas dissolved in a solution is directly proportional to the partial pressure of the gas above that solution. This relationship can be best illustrated by opening a bottle of carbonated drink. As the lid is removed, the partial pressure of gas above the liquid drops sharply, allowing for dissolved carbon dioxide to emerge from the liquid in the form of bubbles. As will be discussed later in this chapter, the most practical significance of Henry's law is in considering the aeromedical transport of a patient at risk of decompression sickness with the drop in atmospheric pressure on ascent, potentially leading to dissolved nitrogen rapidly emerging out of solution from the blood.

2.4   Pathophysiological Consequences of Flight

When we place a patient into an aircraft, whether that be in a fixed- or rotary-wing environment, we need to always consider the potential effects and clinical consequences of:

- Altitude
- Temperature
- Altered humidity
- Acceleration and deceleration
- Noise
- Vibration
- Fatigue and stress

It is important to note that these physiological stressors can have an impact on the aeromedical team as well as the patient. The impact on the flight team is not only physiologic; it can also adversely impact the ability to evaluate the patient.

2.4.1   Effects of Altitude

The most significant effect of altitude is exposure to hypoxia. Hypoxia is defined as a decrease in oxygen availability at the tissue level. Dalton's law tells us that the PiO_2 decreases with increasing altitude, resulting in altitude-induced hypoxia. This is a form of hypoxic hypoxia [5]. You will recall that at sea level, the PiO_2 is 160 mmHg. However, inspired air becomes fully saturated with water vapour as it passes through the upper airways. This process of humidification is very efficient, such that the saturated water vapour pressure (SWVP) of inspired air is a function of temperature only and not altitude. As temperature in the airways is fairly constant, SWVP is also constant across all altitudes at which humans can survive. This equates to 47 mmHg at 37 °C and, therefore, results in an effective PiO_2 at sea level of 0.21 (760 – 47) = 150 mmHg. As it remains constant, the proportional effect of SVWP increases with altitude. For example, at 10,000 ft, it would result in an effective PiO_2 of 0.21 (523 – 47) = 100 mmHg. This issue, along with the elimination of carbon dioxide by the lungs, results in the overall drop in partial pressure of oxygen that occurs from the atmosphere to the alveolus [6]. A further small drop in partial pressure occurs as oxygen is transferred from the alveolus into the arterial circulation. Table 2.3 shows the relationship between altitude and partial pressure of inspired and arterial oxygen.

The hypoxic hypoxia of altitude generally only becomes clinically relevant at altitudes of ~10,000 ft in fit and healthy individuals. However, when transporting sick or injured patients, susceptibility to the effects of altitude-related hypoxia can occur at much lower heights. Why is 10,000 ft such a "magic" number? To understand this phenomenon, we need to review the oxygen-haemoglobin dissociation curve. This curve describes the relationship between the partial pressure of arterial

Table 2.3 Partial pressure of inspired and arterial oxygen with altitude

Altitude ASL (ft)	Atmospheric pressure (mmHg)	PiO_2^a (mmHg) including effects of SVWP	PaO_2^b (mmHG)	SaO_2^c (%)
Sea level	760	150	103	97–100
1,000	733	144	98	
2,000	706	138	94	
3,000	681	133	90	
4,000	656	128	85	
5,000	632	123	81	~94
6,000	609	118	77	
7,000	586	113	73	
8,000	565	109	69	~93
9,000	542	104	65	
10,000	523	100	61	~90

$^a PiO_2$ = partial pressure of inspired oxygen
$^b PaO_2$ = partial pressure of arterial oxygen
$^c SaO_2$ = percentage saturation of haemoglobin with oxygen

Fig. 2.1 Altitude and the oxygen-haemoglobin dissociation curve

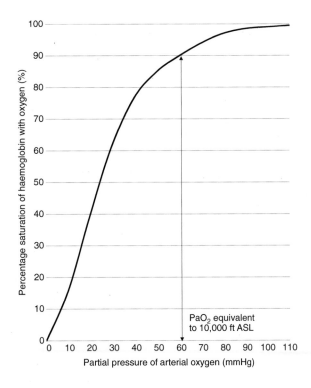

oxygen (PaO_2) and the percentage saturation of haemoglobin with oxygen (SaO_2) [7]. The sigmoid shape of the curve as seen in Fig. 2.1 provides a degree of protection from hypoxia with a significant fall in oxygen saturation not occurring until the PaO_2 falls below ~60 mmHg. Table 2.3 shows us that this level of PaO_2 corresponds with an altitude of ~10,000 ft. This fact explains why most commercial aircraft are able to transport passengers without a resultant physiological compromise whilst pressurised to a cabin altitude of typically between 6,500 and 7,000 ft. At these altitudes, SaO_2 is well maintained above 90%. Note that commercial airlines have a maximum certification cabin altitude of 8,000 ft at the maximum operating altitude of the aircraft that would still allow for adequate oxygen saturation [8].

A question to consider is why commercial airlines do not pressurise their cabins all the way to sea level. The answer relates to engineering considerations rather than medical ones. An aircraft frame is designed to withstand a specific amount of pressure differential between the inside and the outside of the aircraft. At 38,000 ft cruising altitude, with a cabin altitude of 8,000 ft, the typical pressure differential will be approximately 9 psi. If a sea level cabin pressure is maintained all the way to cruising altitude, then the differential pressure would increase as the outside atmospheric pressure falls. This would place ever-greater stresses on the structural integrity of the aircraft, which to overcome would require structural redesign and reinforcement leading to increased overall weight, increased fuel consumption, and operating costs. For commercial airlines, these changes are not economically viable, especially as research has suggested reducing cabin altitude to below 6,000 ft does not offer any meaningful improvement in passenger comfort [9].

Medically, however, there will be clinical scenarios that demand a lower cabin altitude even as far down as sea level. Many dedicated aeromedical aircraft have the capacity to provide this level of pressurisation with a wide range of capabilities existing between different aircraft. It is important, however, to recognise that increasing cabin pressure still has significant aviation implications and that this must, in each case, be weighed against medical need. Some of these considerations include:

- Requirement to operate at a lower cruise altitude
- Limited capacity to fly over bad weather
- Flying at altitudes where turbulence is greater
- Slower air speed

Rotary-wing aircraft, on the other hand, do not have pressurised cabins and patients will essentially be exposed to the surrounding altitude at which the aircraft is operating. The only way to increase cabin pressure is to fly the aircraft at a lower altitude, assuming that it is safe to do so.

The next most significant effect is gas expansion. Boyle's law tells us that the volume of a gas will increase on ascent and decrease on descent [2–4]. Table 2.2 shows us the typical gas expansion ratios at varying altitudes. For example, the volume of gas in an enclosed space at sea level would expand to ~1.2 times its volume at 5,000 ft. The human body contains a large amount of gas in cavities that are either fully or partially closed, such as the middle ear, sinuses, lungs and bowel. Gas expansion in these regions, or in clinical disease states where there is increased accumulation of contained gas, can lead to potentially significant complications. Examples of such conditions include:

- Pneumothorax
- Pneumomediastinum
- Pneumocephalus
- Penetrating eye injury
- Bowel obstruction
- Gas gangrene
- Sinus or middle-ear disease
- Acute decompression sickness
- Post-operative states, involving laparotomy/laparoscopy, thoracotomy, craniotomy, and retinal surgery

The paranasal sinuses offer a good illustration of these effects. The sinuses are air-filled spaces which have fairly rigid walls communicating with the outside world through small orifices known as ostia which open into the nasal cavity. During ascent, the air in the sinus will expand but venting through the ostia will allow the pressure in the sinus to equalise with the cabin pressure. However, conditions such as sinusitis can lead to tissue oedema which can obstruct the ostia and prevent this equalisation from occurring. Now as the air in the sinus expands on ascent, it will lead to increased pressure on the walls of the sinus, resulting in pain.

A pneumothorax is a much-feared condition when flying. Boyle's law predicts that a pneumothorax will expand with increasing altitude, potentially leading to pneumothorax under tension. Whilst gas expansion clearly does occur, there is a degree of controversy in regard to its clinical significance. Whilst the majority of clinicians would not fly a patient with a pneumothorax without first inserting a drain, the true clinical risk of altitude alone on a pneumothorax is unknown. A mathematical model of altitude limitations due to gas expansion has suggested that, at sea level a pneumothorax up to 45% in size may, in fact, be tolerable up to 8,000 ft ASL [10]. Another study placed patients with residual traumatic pneumothorax following the removal of a chest drain into a hypobaric chamber simulating an altitude of greater than 9,000 ft ASL. This found that pneumothorax size increased on average by 5.6 mm from the "pre-flight" chest radiograph, that no patients developed any cardiorespiratory symptoms, and that all had returned to baseline size 4 h "post-flight" [11]. However, many variables influence the management of pneumothorax at any altitude and the body of research in relation to the risks of gas expansion is very small. Note that most commercial airlines will not allow a patient with a pneumothorax to fly until at least 7 days post-confirmation of full expansion [12].

Gas expansion in one region can also impact other organ systems. For example, infants and small children rely on the diaphragm as their principal muscle of respiration. The stomach is full of air and expansion at altitude can lead to gastric dilatation, which can result in diaphragmatic splinting with a dramatic decrease in lung compliance and a drop in functional residual capacity, potentially causing hypoxia, and ultimately respiratory failure. The simple procedure of inserting a nasogastric tube may allow for venting of this air and help to minimise the consequences of this problem [13].

It should also be noted that the contraction of a gas on descent can be as equally problematic as expansion on ascent. The middle ear offers a good illustration. This is another air-filled space that communicates with the outside world through the Eustachian tube. A patent Eustachian tube allows for equalisation to occur between the middle ear and the atmosphere. Conditions such as an upper respiratory tract infection can lead to oedema and obstruction of the tube preventing equalisation. On descent, atmospheric pressure increases in the outer ear but the gas within the middle ear is trapped, resulting in contraction and a decrease in pressure. The widening pressure differential across the tympanic membrane leads to pain and potentially can cause the drum to rupture from the outside inwards. The converse can happen on ascent with trapped air within the middle ear expanding and the increased pressure resulting in a rupture of the tympanic membrane from the inside outwards. Notably, rupture of a tympanic membrane in such circumstances usually results in sudden and dramatic relief of pain as it allows for immediate equalisation [14].

The list above is of examples of gas volume changes occurring inside the body. It should also be noted that hypobaric pressure changes in the air surrounding the body can have a potential impact on tissue pressures. Consider a patient with an extremity fracture. A decrease in the surrounding atmospheric pressure will result in a relative increase in capillary hydrostatic pressure and potentially increase fluid accumulation into the extravascular compartments with worsening oedema. This can be of particular significance in the lower limbs where prolonged immobility in the seated position appears to significantly increase lower leg volume regardless of the presence of injury [15]. The application of a plaster cast where small air bubbles trapped in the plaster can expand further compounds the problem leading to increased external compression. Whilst there is not much direct evidence in regard to the risk of compartment syndrome in such circumstances, most clinicians will advise splitting a plaster cast prior to flying, at least in the first 48 h post-injury.

It is now worth considering scuba diving in the context of the combined effects of both Boyle's and Henry's law. During a dive, the pressure of the surrounding water increases by 1 atmosphere for every 33 ft of descent. This results in increasing amounts of nitrogen dissolving in the blood and accumulating in the lipid component of tissues. During ascent, as the surrounding pressure decreases, nitrogen is released from the tissues back into the blood and from there to the alveoli where it returns to its gaseous form and can participate in respiration. Too rapid an ascent, as predicted by Henry's law, will allow dissolved nitrogen to come out of solution and return to its gaseous form whilst still in the tissues or blood. This allows for the formation of gas bubbles which form the pathophysiological basis of decompression illness. A further problem can occur if flying too soon after a scuba dive. As cabin pressure decreases, subclinical microbubbles can expand, as predicted by Boyle's law, disrupting cells and cellular function if located within the tissues and potentially leading to embolisation if within the blood. It is for this reason that there are defined "no-fly" periods after scuba diving and why patients with decompression illness requiring aeromedical transportation should always be flown at the lowest possible cabin altitude [16]. A review of the literature indicated that no adverse events had been reported during the transport of decompression illness patients if flown at an altitude below 500 ft [17].

Therefore, most clinicians would advocate for a sea level flight in a fixed-wing aircraft and the lowest possible safe altitude in a rotary-wing aircraft.

The effects of changes in gas volume can also impact any medical device with a pneumatic component. Examples include:

- Air-filled splints
- Vacuum mattresses
- Transport ventilators
- Intravenous fluid administration sets
- Endotracheal tube cuffs
- Drainage bags
- Plaster casts

This can be illustrated by considering endotracheal tube cuffs and transport ventilators. An endotracheal tube cuff, being filled with air, can expand on ascent, resulting in increased pressure on the tracheal wall, or contract on descent, increasing the risk of aspiration. One study on endotracheal tube intracuff pressure in 114 patients during helicopter transport showed that with a mean increase in altitude of 2,260 ft, 72% of patients had an intracuff pressure >50 cm H_2O and 20% were >80 cm H_2O. This effect can be overcome by carefully monitoring intracuff pressures, especially during the ascent/descent phases of a flight [18].

Transport ventilators have different design characteristics resulting in some older or less sophisticated models altering their performance at altitude. For example, the Drager Oxylog 1000 has pneumatic logic controls which require a change in gas pressure to trigger a cycle from inspiration to expiration. As altitude increases a larger volume of gas is required to trigger this switch resulting in the delivery of a larger tidal volume than has been set. One study on the performance of Drager Oxylog ventilators showed an increase in delivered minute volume of 11% with the Oxylog 1000 and 15% with the Oxylog 2000 at a simulated altitude of 6,000 ft ASL [19]. More sophisticated ventilators can have a range of pressure sensors and electronic controls to allow for full compensation of any barometric induced change.

2.4.2   Effects of Temperature

Within the physiological zone of the atmosphere there is a temperature drop of ~1–2 °C for every 1,000 ft of ascent. This is not usually a significant issue in most fixed-wing aircraft as there is varying capacity to control the cabin temperature. The greatest flexibility in this regard is when working in a dedicated air ambulance. When transporting a patient on a commercial flight, remember that they have to cater to a wide variety of passengers, with cabin temperature usually set at ~22 +/−2 °C. Most modern commercial aircraft can, however, adjust the temperature across multiple zones allowing for the option to liaise with the crew to try and better optimise the ambient temperature to a patient's needs. The A380, for example, can set cabin temperature between 18 and 30 °C across 15 different temperature control zones [20].

Temperature control can be harder to achieve in rotary-wing airframes and the capacity to do so is very much dependent on the specific platform utilised and the environment in which it is operating. Rotary-wing aircraft can expose both patients and crew to significant variations in temperature. In cold weather, this can lead to heat loss, especially in children or the critically ill patient. Conversely, in hot climates, rotary-wing aircraft can behave like a greenhouse, increasing cabin temperature significantly even at altitude.

Whilst it is important to maintain the thermal integrity of patients during aeromedical transportation, it is important to note that thermal stress can also adversely impact the transport team. Excess heat stress, both hot and cold, can lead to fatigue, decreased attention span, impaired judgement, impaired calculation and poor decision-making, all of which in turn can adversely affect patient care [21].

Medications are also required to be stored at specific temperatures. It is unlikely that many aeromedical services are able to maintain their medications at the correct temperature at all times. Whether the typical fluctuations in temperature that might be encountered in the aviation environment alter medication potency is generally not known. However, it is important to consider the thermal environment in which these operations will occur and to develop storage solutions to maintain as optimal thermal integrity of medications as possible. This is critical in the context of the storage of blood products.

2.4.3   Effects of Altered Humidity

Relative humidity is the ratio of the partial pressure of water vapour in a mixture to the fully saturated water vapour pressure of that mixture at a given temperature. It is an index of how moist the air is. Relative humidity is predominantly a function of temperature and it decreases as the temperature falls. With increasing altitude, there is a progressive fall in temperature and so the relative humidity will also fall. For comfort, humans generally require a relative humidity of between 50 and 70%. This, however, cannot be maintained in aircraft as it would lead to condensation and corrosion and so relative humidity is typically kept in the range of 10–20%. In other words, cabin air while in flight is dry. Generally, the longer the flight time, the lower the average relative humidity will be during that flight.

Prolonged exposure over 3 h or more to this level of relative humidity can lead to drying of the skin and mucosal membranes, which can lead to complications such as sore eyes, sore throat, a dry cough, and epistaxis [22]. Breathing dry air can potentially trigger an exacerbation of COPD or asthma in some susceptible individuals. However, there is no definitive evidence that this level of humidity results in any significant adverse health outcomes in the average passenger. It has also been suggested that breathing dry cabin air leads to an increased number of respiratory tract infections but there is no objective evidence to support this assertion. Despite this, it is appropriate to monitor a patient's hydration status, humidify supplemental oxygen where possible, and protect the corneas from drying out in the patient with altered consciousness.

2.4.4   Effects of Acceleration and Deceleration

Humans have adapted to living life subject to the gravitational force of the Earth. Gravity is an accelerative force acting on objects to change their velocity over unit time. On the surface of the planet, this change is 9.82 m/s^2, referred to as a force of 1G. During flight, the human body can be exposed to either greater or lesser G forces. These can act on the body in a vertical, longitudinal, or lateral axis. G forces are referred to as positive or negative. This does not relate to their intensity but rather the direction of the force. For example, when standing upright, gravity exerts a positive vertical G force. A negative vertical G force would act in the opposite direction of gravity [3, 4].

Furthermore, Newton's third law of motion states that for every action, there is an equal and opposite reaction. When an object accelerates or decelerates in one direction, there will therefore be an equal force applied in the opposite direction, referred to as an inertial force. In relation to G forces and Newton's third law, the most significant impact of flight is on the circulatory system. Consider a patient lying on a stretcher with their head to the front of a fixed-wing aircraft. As the aircraft accelerates for take-off, the patient will be exposed to positive G forces. This will result in the inertial force acting in the opposite direction, increasing blood flow away from the brain and towards the feet. The opposite will occur on landing. The physiological response to these forces will depend on their direction, duration, and intensity. Positive G forces, which increase blood flow away from the brain, are better tolerated than negative G forces, which increase blood flow into the brain [23]. Healthy individuals can compensate for short-term changes in blood flow, but there may be potentially adverse consequences in the critically ill patient with haemodynamic and/or neurological compromise. For example, venous pooling in the legs may exacerbate hypotension in the haemodynamically-compromised patient with conditions such as sepsis or blood loss, and lead to a decrease in cerebral perfusion. Conversely, increased blood flow to the brain may lead to an increase in intracranial pressure, which may be clinically significant in neurologically compromised patients, such as those with head injury.

Humans can potentially tolerate very-short-term exposure to positive G forces of up to ~9G, although most will lose consciousness with sustained exposure of ~4G. Light-sensitive retinal cells are very sensitive to decreased perfusion and so greying of vision followed by complete loss of vision will often precede loss of consciousness. However, tolerance to negative G forces is much more limited to ~2–3G before losing consciousness as a result of marked intracranial pooling of blood. The forces patients are usually exposed to in aeromedical operations are small and generally within the range of 1G +/−0.25G, although turbulence or the need to undertake sudden manoeuvres can lead to greater short-term changes [23]. There is no good evidence to substantiate the direct clinical impact of these changes in the real-world retrieval environment, but it is prudent to always consider the potential impact of G forces on critically ill patients and take those into account when considering the optimum positioning of the patient in the selected transport platform.

2.4.5   Effects of Noise

The aeromedical environment is noisy. Ambient noise varies according to the aircraft type and specific phase of flight. Noise levels in a typical commercial aircraft can vary throughout the flight from ~65 to 85 dBA, whereas in turboprop or rotary-wing aircraft, this can exceed 95dBA. Typical noise exposure standards indicate that an exposure of 85 dBA averaged over an 8 h period is the acceptable upper limit to avoid damage to hearing. Note that every 3 dBA increase in noise is equivalent to a doubling of energy output and thus a halving of the acceptable exposure time. Therefore, exposure to 88 dBA averaged over 4 h or 91 dBA averaged over 2 h would be equivalent to the 85 dBA over 8-h standard. For comparison, normal conversation occurs at ~20 dBA.

Exposure to noise has a significant impact on individuals [24, 25]. Apart from the potential for hearing loss, human performance appears to be adversely influenced by exposure to both sustained and intermittent noise. This can lead to fatigue, irritability, impaired cognition, and compromised ability to perform tasks. The main impact appears to be with complex tasks where prolonged concentration is required, such as the clinical management of a patient in flight. It should be noted that there is a great degree of inter-individual variation in the tolerance to noise, which is influenced by an individual's state of arousal, personality, motivation, and prior experience. It has also been noted that the performance of simple repetitive tasks may in fact be enhanced by noise. Aircraft noise can of course also impair communication between members of the retrieval team and the patient, which can compromise safety and lead to both clinical and operational errors.

The physiological and psychological impact of noise on a patient is unclear. It can lead to sleep deprivation in the critically ill patient, which in turn can contribute to cardiovascular stress, impaired immunity and catabolic metabolism. Noise also increases sedation and analgesia requirements in the critically ill. Exposure to noise may lead to fear, anxiety, and stress which in part may predispose to the development of confusion, delirium, and psychosis. It is important to always consider the impact of noise on both the retrieval team and the patient and to take steps to minimise its impact through the use of aids such as ear plugs and headphones.

2.4.6   Effects of Vibration

Vibration is defined as periodic oscillation in relation to a fixed equilibrium point. Organs, organ systems, and the body in general all have their own natural frequency of vibration [26]. External vibrations close to these natural frequencies will result in amplification of vibration. Typical body resonant frequencies are:

- Shoulder girdle 4–5 Hz
- Abdominal organs 4–8 Hz
- Head 5–6 Hz
- Facial tissues 15–20 Hz

- Eyes 60–90 Hz
- Whole body (vertical plane) 2–10 Hz
- Whole body (horizontal plane) less than 3 Hz

Flight can increase exposure to vibration [3, 4]. This can be from sources within the aircraft, such as the engine, or external to the aircraft, such as turbulent air. In a rotary-wing aircraft, vibration occurs in all axes of movement and is generally worse in the transition stages to hover. Rotating components and gears are the main sources of vibration in rotary-wing aircraft, whereas engine operation, propellers, and turbulence are the principal sources related to fixed-wing aircraft. Transmission of vibration to the body can have a number of adverse events [27]. These include generalised discomfort and fatigue from muscle contractions in an attempt to dampen the vibration and low back pain especially for those in a seated position. There can be impairment of capacity to undertake precise manual tasks by vibration at frequencies of ~4–6 Hz and blurring of vision can occur at frequencies of 2–20 Hz. Speech can be distorted at frequencies of 4–12 Hz and prolonged exposure to vibration can impair the ability to undertake complex cognitive tasks. Low-frequency oscillations provoke motion sickness. These can be up to ~0.7 Hz with maximum nausea potential being around 0.2 Hz [28]. These effects can be particularly significant for retrieval teams that work constantly within the aeromedical environment and can be a significant contributor to fatigue, impairment of the ability to perform complex cognitive tasks, and subsequent human error.

In patients with haemorrhage, such as those with major pelvic trauma, vibrations may potentially destabilise clots and facilitate increased bleeding [29]. Some clinicians believe that vibration may impact adversely the cardiovascular and respiratory systems. There is also a theoretical risk of increased bubble formation in patients with decompression illness. Tribonucleation is a physical process where gas bubbles can be formed at an interface where two adherent surfaces are rapidly pulled apart. Vibration appears to accelerate this process, although its impact in vivo is not known [30]. Indeed, the overall risks to a patient in relation to vibration are not well understood and the complex characteristics of vibration in the aeromedical environment make it very difficult to conduct meaningful research in this area. However, it is still important to remain alert to the actual and potential effects of vibration on both aircrew and patients and to attempt to reduce those effects where possible. This is primarily an engineering issue relating to areas such as stretcher design, restraint systems, damping mechanisms, and overall aircraft maintenance. Finally, be aware that vibration can also impact medical equipment either by affecting its function, such as with non-invasive oscillometric blood pressure monitors and activity-sensing pacemakers, or by leading to dislodgement, such as the migration of an endotracheal tube.

2.4.7 Effects of Fatigue and Stress

This is primarily a concern for the aircrew. Factors inherent to the flight environment that increase fatigue include:

- Hypoxia
- Thermal stress
- Noise
- Vibration
- Dehydration
- Physical activity
- Increased workload
- Motion sickness

Fatigue, in turn, leads to a lack of motivation, impaired short-term memory, increased reaction time, impaired judgement, intolerance, frustration, risk-taking behaviour, and poor decision-making. In other words, fatigue leads to mistakes [31]. None of these traits are helpful in the conduct of a complex medical repatriation.

2.4.8 Motion Sickness

Motion sickness is caused by exposure to actual or apparent motion that you are unfamiliar with. The pathophysiology is complex and not fully understood, but it is essentially the result of a conflict of sensory inputs between what your eyes see, what your vestibular apparatus senses, and what signals your brain expects as opposed to those it actually receives. The motion associated with flight can commonly lead to motion sickness, particularly in turbulent conditions, as your inability to fully visualise the outside world whilst the aircraft is moving can lead to such a vestibular-visual conflict. The most important thing to remember in regard to motion sickness is that it can affect anyone at any time, including aircrew who have flown extensively with no prior problems. Pregnant individuals, children, people with prior or current vestibular disease, migraine sufferers, and those who exhibit marked anxiety about the potential for motion sickness appear are at increased risk. General malaise, sweating, nausea, vomiting, and an exaggerated sense of motion are typical features. Malaise, lethargy, and fatigue can persist for many hours [32]. This can not only be unpleasant, but if occurring in the aircrew can also significantly compromise their ability to carry out their essential functions.

2.5 Summary

There are many significant physiological consequences and environmental stressors in relation to the transport of a patient in a hypobaric aviation environment. It is important to understand the implications of these on normal human physiology and what steps can be taken to minimise the potential for related adverse clinical consequences in sick or injured patients being transported by air. It is equally important to remember that these physiological changes and environmental stressors can impact the aircrew and medical equipment. Finally, it is worth noting that whilst the potential implications of these changes are generally well understood, their actual clinical significance is not. For example, Boyle's law clearly predicts that a pneumothorax will expand at altitude, but does that mean that there is a risk of clinical deterioration or even tension when we fly such a patient, and if so, is it likely also dependent on other factors such as the aetiology of the pneumothorax, duration of flight, and associated comorbidities? Unfortunately, the relatively isolated and potentially hostile nature of the aeromedical environment is a difficult one in which to establish high-quality clinical trials and most such questions have not been, and indeed may never be, answered by research.

References

1. Gratton G. The atmosphere. In: Gratton G, editor. Initial airworthiness: determining the acceptability of new airborne systems. Switzerland: Springer; 2015. p. 15–32.
2. Reinhart RO. Basic flight physiology. 3rd ed. New York: McGraw-Hill; 2008.
3. Martin T. Aeromedical Transportation: a clinical guide. 2nd ed. Aldershot: Ashgate; 2006.
4. Grissom T. Critical care air transport: patient flight physiology and organizational considerations. In: Hurd WW, Jernigan JG, editors. Aeromedical evacuation: management of acute and stabilized patients. New York: Springer; 2003. p. 111–35.
5. Wirth D, Rumberger E. Fundamentals of aviation physiology. In: Christiansen CC, Draeger J, Kriebel J, editors. Principles and practice of aviation medicine. New Jersey: World Scientific; 2009. p. 71–150.
6. West JB, Schoene RB, Luks AM, Milledge JS. The atmosphere. In: High altitude medicine and physiology. 5th ed. Boca Raton: CRC Press; 2013. p. 16–27.
7. West JB. Respiratory physiology: the essentials. 9th ed. Baltimore: Lippincott Williams & Wilkins; 2012.
8. Aerospace Medical Association, Aviation Safety Committee, Civil Aviation Subcommittee. Cabin cruising altitudes for regular transport aircraft. Aviat Space Environ Med. 2008;79(4):433–9.
9. Muhm JM, Rock PB, McMullin DL, Jones SP, Lu IL, Eilers KD, et al. Effect of aircraft-cabin altitude on passenger discomfort. N Engl J Med. 2007;357:18–27.
10. Fitz-Clark J, Quinlan D, Valani R. Flying with a pneumothorax: a model of altitude limitations due to gas expansion. Aviat Space Environ Med. 2013;84(8):834–9.
11. Majercik S, White TW, Van Boerum DH, Granger S, Bledsoe J, Conner K, et al. Cleared for takeoff: the effects of hypobaric conditions on traumatic pneumothoraces. J Trauma Acute Care Surg. 2014;77(5):729–33.
12. International Air Transport Association. Medical manual. 8th ed. 2016 [cited 2016 Nov 23]. http://www.iata.org/publications/Pages/medical-manual.aspx.
13. Samuels MP. The effects of flight and altitude. Arch Dis Child. 2004;89:448–55.
14. Kanick SC, Doyle WJ. Barotrauma during air travel: predictions of a mathematical model. J Appl Physiol. 2005;98(5):1592–602.
15. Mittermayr M, Fries D, Gruber H, Peer S, Klingler A, Fischbach U, et al. Leg edema formation and venous blood flow velocity during a simulated long-haul flight. Thromb Res. 2007;120(4):497–504.
16. Stephenson J. Pathophysiology, treatment and aeromedical retrieval of SCUBA-related DCI. J Mil Veterans Health. 2009;17(3):10–9.
17. MacDonald RD, O'Donnell C, Allen B, Breeck K, Chow Y, DeMajo W, et al. Interfacility transport of patients with decompression illness: literature review and consensus statement. Prehosp Emerg Care. 2006;10:482–7.
18. Bassi M, Zuercher M, Erne JJ, Ummenhofer W. Endotracheal tube intracuff pressure duriung helicopter transport. Ann Emerg Med. 2010;56(2):89–93.
19. Flynn JG, Singh B. The performance of Drager Oxylog ventilators at simulated altitude. Anaesth Intensive Care. 2008;36:549–52.
20. Dechow M, Nurcombe CAH. Aircraft environmental control systems. In: Hocking MB, editor. Air quality in airplane cabins and similar enclosed spaces. New York: Springer; 2005. p. 4–24.

21. Pilcher JJ, Nadler E, Busch C. Effects of hot and cold temperature exposure on performance: a meta-analytic review. Ergonomics. 2002;45(10):682–98.
22. Nagda NL, Hodgson M. Low relative humidity and aircraft cabin air quality. Indoor Air. 2001;11(3):200–14.
23. Newman DG. High G flight: physiological effects and countermeasures. Farnham: Ashgate; 2015.
24. Metidieri MM, Rodrigues HFS, Barros de Oliveira Filho FJM, Ferraz DP, Fausto de Almeida Neto A, Torres S. Noise induced hearing loss (NIHL): literature review with a focus on occupational medicine. Int Arch Otorhinolaryngol. 2013;17(2):208–12.
25. Nassiri P, Monazam M, Fouladi Dehaghi B, et al. The effect of noise on human performance: A clinical trial. Int J Occup Environ Med. 2013;4:87–95.
26. Randall JM, Matthews RT, Stiles MA. Resonant frequencies of standing humans. Ergonomics. 1997;40(9):879–86.
27. Griffin MJ. Handbook of human vibration. London: Academic Press; 1990.
28. Golding JF, Mueller AG, Gresty MA. A motion sickness maximum around the 0.2 Hz frequency range of horizontal translational oscillation. Aviat Space Enviro Med. 2001;72(3):188–92.
29. Carchietti E, Cecchi A, Valent F, Rammer R. Flight vibrations and bleeding in helicoptered patients with pelvic fractures. Air Med J. 2013;32(2):80–3.
30. Vann RD, Clark HG. Bubble growth and mechanical properties of tissue in decompression. Undersea Biomed Res. 1975;2(3):185–94.
31. Lockley SW, Bargar LK, Ayas NT, Rothschild JM, Czeisler CA, Landrigan CP. Effects of health care provider work hours and sleep deprivation on safety and performance. Jt Comm J Qual Patient Saf. 2007;33(11 Suppl 1):S7–18.
32. Brainard A, Gresham C. Motion sickness clinical presentation [Internet]. New York: Medscape; 2016. [cited 2016 Dec 1]. http://emedicine.medscape.com/article/2060606-clinical

Medicolegal Issues Arising from In-Flight Medical Emergencies in Commercial Travel

3

J. Gregory Webb and E. Kyle McNew

3.1 Introduction

This chapter discusses the legal issues and implications surrounding the provision of medical care during a commercial flight. Those issues primarily concern what and whose law governs the situation, and the resulting liability implications and protections for physicians and other healthcare providers. The first section addresses the Aviation Medical Assistance Act and the parameters it sets forth for protecting air carriers and healthcare providers. This section also addresses how healthcare provider liability might be addressed under the Act, depending upon the state in which a claim is pursued. International carrier liability is briefly discussed, but given the fact that there is no uniform liability standard, it is difficult to predict how such actions may resolve. In-flight medical encounters are addressed in the next section, which concludes that there is insufficient data compiled by the government and carriers to effectively analyze it, but there is enough to know that there are tens of thousands of medical incidents each year, making it a real possibility that a healthcare provider could be confronted with such an event during commercial air travel. Lastly, the chapter addresses important considerations before giving care, such as there is no actual legal requirement to begin giving medical care during a commercial flight, but if care is begun, the provider must satisfy general requirements as detailed below.

3.2 The Aviation Medical Assistance Act

In the middle and late 1990s, the United States Government and the aviation industry began to focus on in-flight medical emergencies, with a specific focus on cardiac emergencies. Some, but not all, airlines had already equipped certain of their flights

J. Gregory Webb, Esq. (✉) • E. Kyle McNew, Esq.
MichieHamlett PLLC (Attorneys at Law), Charlottesville, VA, USA
e-mail: GWebb@michiehamlett.com; KMcNew@michiehamlett.com

© Springer International Publishing AG, part of Springer Nature 2018
J. V. Nable, W. Brady (eds.), *In-Flight Medical Emergencies*,
https://doi.org/10.1007/978-3-319-74234-2_3

25

with automatic external defibrillators (AED). Congress held hearings throughout 1997 on the deployment of AEDs on commercial airlines, and several additional airlines began voluntarily equipping certain of their flights with AEDs. Congressional reports produced during this inquiry observed that "the most commonly observed serious in-flight medical events are cardiac in nature, with ventricular fibrillation being the most common form of abnormal heart rhythm" [1].

In 1998, Congress passed the Aviation Medical Assistance Act of 1998 ("Act") [2]. Notably, the Act extends only to "air carriers," which are defined as US companies [2]. Thus, the Act does not apply to foreign air carriers, even those flying into and out of US airports [3].

The Act is primarily a directive from Congress to the Federal Aviation Administration ("FAA") to evaluate and, if appropriate, issue regulations governing what is necessary in the medical kits aboard commercial airliners, specifically whether AEDs must be included, and the training of flight attendants in the use of that equipment [2]. The Act also addresses requirements that major air carriers report certain details of deaths that occur on their flights or as a result of in-flight incidents [2].

The FAA conducted the required evaluation and eventually promulgated regulations concerning the required medical equipment and training. Those regulations currently state that all flights for which a flight attendant is required must contain at least one approved emergency medical kit (see Table 1.1 for items currently required in approved medical kits) [4]. Then, all aircraft for which a flight attendant is required and a maximum payload capacity greater than 7,500 pounds must also contain an AED [4]. This directive translates to aircraft with a capacity of approximately 30 passengers. Thus, certain very small commuter flights may not have AEDs on board.

The final substantive section of the Act creates two different limitations on liability. First, for the airline, the Act imposes a very high barrier to liability for its role in seeking to obtain assistance from passengers to address an in-flight medical emergency:

> An air carrier shall not be liable for damages in any action brought in a Federal or State court arising out of the performance of the air carrier in obtaining or attempting to obtain the assistance of a passenger in an in-flight medical emergency, or out of the acts or omissions of the passenger rendering the assistance, if the passenger is not an employee or agent of the carrier and the carrier in good faith believes that the passenger is a medically qualified individual [2].

As long as the passenger is not an employee or agent of the airline and the airline has a good faith belief that the passenger is a "medically qualified individual," which is defined as "any person who is licensed, certified, or otherwise qualified to provide medical care in a State, including a physician, nurse, physician assistant, paramedic, and emergency medical technician" [2], the airline is completely immune from liability related to passengers who assist during an in-flight emergency.

The second limitation on liability in the Act applies to passengers—such as doctors, nurses, and EMTs—who provide assistance during an in-flight emergency:

An individual shall not be liable for damages in any action brought in a Federal or State court arising out of the acts or omissions of the individual in providing or attempting to provide assistance in the case of an in-flight medical emergency unless the individual, while rendering such assistance, is guilty of gross negligence or willful misconduct [2].

This subsection does not explicitly state that it protects only individuals aboard "air carriers," i.e., US airliners, so it is perhaps arguable that it protects anyone in flight in the United States regardless of what flag the aircraft flies. However, given that the rest of the Act is limited to "air carriers," it is likely that this specific limitation of liability also applies only to individuals aboard an "air carrier's" airplane.

This subsection does not create complete immunity. Instead, it is a qualified immunity from liability that can be overcome by a showing of "gross negligence" or "willful misconduct." This begs the question of what qualifies as "gross negligence" and "willful misconduct." Somewhat surprisingly, as of this writing, there are no reported decisions applying the Act to a claim against a passenger (e.g., physician, nurse) for treatment provided by the passenger during an in-flight emergency, so there is no guidance in the case law about the meaning of "gross negligence" or "willful misconduct." Moreover, those terms are not defined in the Act itself, there is not any definition from some other source referenced in the Act, and there is not any uniform definition of those terms for purposes of federal law. It is worth noting, however, that under the Act, those providing medical assistance aboard a commercial airliner must be medically qualified to do so and cannot be paid for the care provided [2]. There are a handful of reported decisions discussing the Act's applicability to claims against the airline, but no decisions applying the limitation of liability in § 5(b) of the Act. The closest is *Baillie v. MedAire, Inc.*, No. 14-cv-420, 2015 U.S. Dist. LEXIS 164350 (D. Az. Dec. 8, 2015), in which a federal court in Arizona ruled that the § 5(b) limitation of liability did not protect doctors or nurses employed by a company who contracts with airliners to provide medical and treatment advice over the phone to flight crews while a flight is in the air. Even though the text of § 5(b) speaks in terms of any individual involved with providing assistance during an in-flight medical emergency, and could thus be construed to include even individuals who are not passengers on the flight itself, the court ruled that the context of the Act indicates that the § 5(b) protection is intended solely for passengers on the plane who volunteer to help, not individuals who are involved in return for monetary compensation.

"Gross negligence," and to a lesser extent "willful misconduct," is a concept typically found in tort law, which is primarily a creature of state law. Generally speaking, many states adhere to three basic standards of negligence, listed in increasing severity: (1) "simple" or "ordinary" negligence; (2) "gross" negligence; and (3) "willful" or "willful and wanton" negligence. There is very little federal tort law on the latter. Thus, it makes some sense that these terms are undefined for purposes of the Act, but it is nevertheless problematic because the concepts also have no uniform definition from state to state. Though everyone can generally agree that "gross negligence" is something more than simple negligence, Massachusetts may define "gross negligence" slightly differently than Virginia, Illinois, and/or Texas.

Assume that a doctor from Virginia boards a flight in Boston, bound for Los Angeles. The airline has its corporate headquarters in Delaware. Somewhere over Kansas, a passenger begins experiencing chest pains. The doctor responds to the crew's request that any doctor aboard identify himself/herself, and provides treatment to the passenger. The passenger thereafter sues the doctor for medical malpractice. Because the Act applies to this situation, the passenger will have to allege and prove that the doctor was at least grossly negligent in the treatment provided during the flight. But whose definition of gross negligence will govern that inquiry? The passenger could probably bring suit in Massachusetts, Kansas, Virginia, Delaware, or California. Each of those states will have its own definition of "gross negligence" as well as its own choice of law rules for determining which state's definition will govern. Thus, a court in Virginia may determine that Kansas or Massachusetts law applies, and use that state's definition of gross negligence.

It is impossible to predict how this question would be resolved in any given case because the analysis is so fact intensive. Moreover, the definitional differences may not be all that important because those differences from state to state tend to be marginal and nuanced. Thus, one state's definition of "gross negligence" is not likely to include or exclude many fact patterns that would not also be included or excluded by another state's definition. The fact remains, however, that in any case in which qualified immunity is at issue under § 5(b) of the Aviation Medical Assistance Act, there likely will be a legal battle over which state law applies and what gross negligence means. If such a case arose, lawyers representing the injured party would likely look at which state or jurisdiction had the most favorable tort law for alleged victims of medical negligence. Variables that would be examined would be the jurisdiction's restrictions on damages (such as noneconomic damage caps), the state's laws on contributory or comparative negligence, and how receptive the particular venue in the state might be to such a claim.

The same issues exist for "willful misconduct" as used in § 5(b) of the Act. "Gross negligence" is a phrase and concept found in virtually every state's jurisprudence. However, "willful misconduct" as a liability standard is not. For example, some states have a concept called "willful and wanton negligence," which may be synonymous with "willful misconduct." Or it may not be. "Willful misconduct" could be closer conceptually to intentional torts like battery. Thus, as with gross negligence, an in-flight emergency case that alleges "willful misconduct" will first involve a dispute to define what that means. That being said, given that there are no reported decisions involving a gross negligence claim under the Act, a case implicating the "willful misconduct" standard under the Act will be even rarer still.

In sum, the sheer lack of reported decisions involving § 5(b) of the Act suggests that the requirement of proving at least "gross negligence" is a significant deterrent to any potential plaintiff contemplating a claim against a volunteer responding to an in-flight medical emergency. This makes intuitive sense. Despite varying slightly from state to state, "gross negligence" has historically been defined in terms of acting without even slight care [5]. It would take very compelling facts to reconcile the notion of a medical provider volunteering to assist a fellow passenger during an in-flight medical emergency with the notion of acting without even slight care.

Thus, given the limitation of liability in § 5(b) of the Act, healthcare professionals aboard domestic flights should have a relatively high degree of confidence that saying "yes" when a flight attendant comes over the intercom asking if there is a doctor or nurse aboard is unlikely to be inviting liability for medical malpractice. Lastly, but importantly, the optics of suing a physician rendering "Good Samaritan" aid to a patient in need are not appealing to most experienced trial attorneys.

3.3   The Montreal Convention: International Carriers

As stated above, the Aviation Medical Assistance Act applies only to "air carriers"—airlines based in the United States. It is unclear whether the protections of the Act extend to air carriers operating internationally, such as a Delta flight from Atlanta to Rome. Because there is nothing in the Act saying that the Act would not apply in such a situation, it is likely that the Act would apply in litigation brought in the United States.

Regardless of the nationality of the carrier, virtually all international flights are also governed by the Convention for the Unification of Certain Rules for International Carriage by Air, commonly referred to as the "Montreal Convention." The Montreal Convention was signed in 1999 and became effective in 2003, and supplanted the prior "Warsaw Convention." The Montreal Convention has been ratified by 119 countries and the European Union.

The Montreal Convention deals exclusively with the relationship and liabilities between customer and carrier. It has no "Good Samaritan" provision analogous to § 5(b) of the Aviation Medical Assistance Act that would provide any sort of protection or limitation of liability to third-party passengers such as a volunteer doctor. Accordingly, on many international flights, and on all flights by international carriers, there is no uniformly applicable liability standard for volunteer healthcare providers during an in-flight medical emergency. Those standards would, instead, be determined by the substantive law and choice of law rules of the country in which litigation is maintained.

3.4   In-Flight Medical Encounters

While in-flight medical incidents are relatively common, they are not commonly reported or studied [6]. The reasons are obvious given the environment, the relatively short time periods involved, and the transfer of care that takes place once the aircraft lands. Thus, other than the Act discussed above, and whatever state law may apply given the choice of law, there are essentially no other guidelines in place for healthcare practitioners who find themselves in flight and asked to render health care.

Further, as one would expect given the above, there is no uniform system set up by federal or state authorities to monitor the incidence of in-flight medical emergencies. Thus, analyzing, comparing, and making recommendations based upon the data are speculative.

We do know that "MedAire, a medical assistance company that provides remote assistance to several commercial airlines in the United States, responds to an average of 17,000 cases per year" [6]. It is still difficult to extrapolate that number to the entire number of incidents involving all domestic airlines. But, suffice it to say the numbers appear to be well into the tens of thousands of in-flight medical incidents per year. Given these numbers, as a healthcare provider traveling on a commercial flight, the possibility of being called upon to render medical assistance is quite real and should be considered before boarding a commercial aircraft.

3.5   Important Considerations Before Giving Care

Notwithstanding the above, first and foremost, as in any other situation, there is no legal requirement for a healthcare provider to intervene or get involved with an in-flight emergency. In most jurisdictions, absent some sort of legally defined "special relationship," the law imposes no duty upon anyone to act in aid of another, which extends to any licensed medical provider, including physicians, nurses, physician assistants, paramedics, and emergency medical technicians. Thus, absent some "special relationship" (e.g., the sick individual is a current patient; or the physician begins administering care and then stops during the flight), a physician can refuse to become involved during such a flight. Whether there is an ethical requirement of involvement is beyond the scope of this chapter, but there can be no legal liability for abstaining from involvement.

The legal regimes discussed above also do not reach or alter any sort of documentation requirement specific to the volunteer healthcare provider. Generally, physicians volunteering to assist during in-flight emergencies (a) should be knowledgeable about the most common in-flight medical problems; (b) should know or find out what medical equipment is aboard the aircraft that could assist the physician; (c) should coordinate the care with the flight crew and those assisting from the ground; and (d) should only provide care within their training, experience, ability, licensing, and scope of practice [6].

Thus, the provider should attempt to adhere to the standard of care applicable in his or her licensing jurisdiction when it comes to documenting an encounter during an in-flight medical emergency. If the practitioner embarks upon care of a passenger in need of medical assistance, then he or she will likely be held to the standard of care governing the specific medical problem or medical specialty dictating the event. This can most easily be accomplished by filling out an incident report with the airline. However, even if the provider fails to document the encounter, any liability arising out of that failure would still be subject to § 5(b)'s (Liability Limitations under the Act) requirement of proving at least gross negligence. And, as discussed above, that is very high hurdle. Notwithstanding the substantial legal challenges for a passenger inclined to pursue a medical negligence claim or lawsuit, it is prudent for the medical provider to document or chart the in-flight encounter in the same manner the provider is accustomed to doing in his or her professional life. The reasons for this are the same as those that apply to the provider's practice.

Conclusion

As the brevity of this chapter suggests, the medicolegal issues surrounding in-flight medical emergencies are not particularly complex. Nor is there an abundance of medical encounters or incidents to study in the United States. While the possibility of the healthcare professional encountering an in-flight medical emergency is low, the likelihood of incurring any kind of liability for volunteering to provide in-flight medical treatment is even lower due to the heightened liability standard provided by the Aviation Medical Assistance Act. This assumes, of course, that the physician rendering care is doing so within the scope of his or her education, training, and experience.

References

1. Stone v. Frontier Airlines, Inc., 256 F. Supp. 2d 29, 33-34 (D. Mass. 2002).
2. Pub. L. No. 105-170, 112 Stat. 47.
3. See, e.g. Horvath v. Deutsche Lufthansa, AG, No. 02-cv-3269, 2004 U.S. Dist. LEXIS 3873, at *3 (S.D.N.Y. Mar. 12, 2004) (observing that the Act does not apply to "foreign carriers are excluded from its reach").
4. 14. C.F.R. § 121.803.
5. Black's Law Dictionary 1057 (7th ed. 1999); William L. Prosser, Handbook of the Law of Torts § 34 (4th ed. 1971).
6. Chandra A, Conroy S. Inflight medical emergencies. West J Emerg Med. 2013;14:499–504.

International Flight Considerations

4

Terrence Mulligan

4.1 Introduction

In the last 20 years, the number of passengers traveling on planes has increased exponentially. The International Civil Aviation Organization (ICAO) along with other sources reports the number of persons traveling by air to be more than 2.5–3.2 billion worldwide every year, with an estimated 5% of travelers experiencing a chronic illness [1–4]. Although air travel is quite safe from a technical point of view, passengers are increasingly at risk during flight due to individual health problems [5]. Although air travel is growing safer and more comfortable, the increasing average age of passengers, heightened security, and stress surrounding flights and schedules, combined with the unique environment of airplanes with changes in cabin temperature, air pressure and humidity levels, narrow seats, and frequent flight delays, may result in adverse medical conditions during flights [6]. Combined with the rising number of passengers and increased capacity of larger aircraft with more long-distance domestic and international flights [2, 7], with long-haul aircrafts—such as the Airbus A380 and Boeing 777 LR now capable of extending flight times to 18–20 h—it is likely that the incidence of in-flight medical emergencies will continue to increase in the coming years [3]. International air travel in particular combines long-haul, extended flight times with unique exposures, and an even more austere, secluded environment for passengers with acute and/or chronic illnesses, and suggests unique medical challenges for recognition, stabilization, treatment, diagnosis, and disposition.

T. Mulligan, D.O., M.P.H.
Department of Emergency Medicine, University of Maryland School of Medicine, Baltimore, MD, USA

4.2   Background

As the population ages, the number of travelers with health problems is also likely to increase, which may lead to an increase in the number of in-flight medical emergencies. Although they are uncommon, medical emergencies do happen on airplanes in flight [8]. Certain examples in the literature indicate that urgent medical conditions during flights have increased gradually [6].

Although the actual number of medical emergencies occurring in flight is unknown due to difficulties and lack of standardization in reporting, it is estimated that between 1 in 10,000 and 1 in 40,000 passengers per year will experience a medical emergency in flight [9]. In recent studies, urgent medical and surgical situations during air travel have been reported as 10–40 demands per 100,000 passengers [2, 5, 10–12]. Data from research studies conducted during the last few years have shown significant increases in in-flight medical emergencies (IMEs) worldwide, but data and knowledge on the incidences, causes, and consequences are still limited, nonuniform, and difficult to gather [3, 5, 7, 13, 14].

Although a majority of in-flight medical incidents are minor, as many as 7–13% of medical emergencies result in aircraft diversion or unscheduled emergency landing [11]. In-flight deaths are quite rare, with an estimated rate of only 0.3–1 death per million passengers per year [9]. The most common reason for a diversion is a cardiac event [15]. Diversions can be quite costly for an airline, with cost estimates ranging from $30,000 to more than $725,000, depending on the situation [15]. These figures do not include the additional costs to other passengers of missed connecting flights and other delays [8].

Qureshi and Porter, in their study of one major international air carrier, found that in 75% of medical emergencies either a doctor or a nurse responded to the air crew's request for help, and 11% of the time a paramedic responded with assistance [7]. A study by the Medlink group (a ground-based medical consulting service for airlines) found a similar rate of response, with medical professionals responding to in-flight medical emergencies about 70% of the time [8, 16]. However, in one study, in the year ending 31 March 1999, British Airways carried 36.8 million passengers and there were 3,386 reported in-flight medical incidents: about 1 per 11,000 passengers. Although 70% were managed by cabin crew without the assistance of an onboard health professional, in almost 1,000 incidents doctors and nurses were asked to help with the management of ill passengers [17].

4.3   Differences in Medical Emergencies on International Flights

Estimating the frequency of in-flight medical events is challenging because no mandatory reporting system exists [17]. Various prevalence data sources exist but most have been derived from individual airlines. In 1999, British Airways reported about one in-flight medical incident per 11,000 passengers [18]. A 2000 UK Government report indicated that the number can be as high as 1 in 1,400 passengers, and a study of a ground-based communications center that provides medical consultative service to airlines estimated that medical emergencies occur in 1 of every 604 flights [4, 17]. Estimates of medical events requiring professional intervention were thought to be about 1 per 14,000 passengers [19].

These data are an average of short-haul and long-haul flights; given the reduced time on the plane with short-haul flights, and the decreased likelihood of passengers seeking help when they are closer to their destination, medical events are likely to be higher than this estimate on long-haul, international flights. In most cases, the incidence of IMEs is likely to increase with the continued growth in air travel, with the gradual aging of the traveling population, and with people with preexisting disease traveling by air, and as airlines continue to reduce prices by reducing seat sizes and increasing passenger numbers [20].

Providing medical care with limited resources, space, support personnel, and equipment creates a suboptimal environment for those physicians, nurses, and other medical professionals who often are asked to volunteer to provide care. Furthermore, some physicians may be reluctant to volunteer to assist in such emergencies given the current litigious environment [21]. The reliance of airlines on volunteer medical assistance combines with several other issues: inadequate space and seating for passengers, inadequate space to provide proper and adequate medical care, inadequate training of crew members, inadequate medical equipment, and inadequate or unclear laws pertaining to volunteer providers, crew members, airlines, and patients, especially on international flights crossing state and national borders and airline ownership; all these combine to increase difficulties of medical stabilization, treatment, diagnosis, and disposition, and even more so on long-haul, international flights [21].

4.4 General Medical Conditions Affected by Long-Haul International Flights

The unique environments associated with aviation, inside and outside the cabin, combined with passenger-specific preexisting medical conditions and risk factors, plus the suboptimal conditions for medical care, diagnosis, and treatment on long-haul flights, all result in increased medical risk for passengers, and likely increased in-flight emergencies on long-haul, international flights.

Exacerbation of preexisting medical problems such as respiratory or cardiovascular conditions can create medical emergencies in the air if passengers do not disclose pertinent information or their treating physicians do not fully understand the risks of flight. In addition, newly presenting medical conditions (e.g., syncope or dyspnea) may also manifest themselves at altitude. Such events may be presumed to be worst-case scenarios (e.g., syncope could be a manifestation of lethal arrhythmias, abdominal aortic aneurysm, or ruptured ectopic pregnancy) [22].

The special environments associated with aviation, reduced atmospheric pressure, reduced available oxygen, increased noise and vibration, and external subfreezing temperatures, can place certain patients at increased risk for medical emergencies.

The cabin environment itself contributes to specific medical risks, which are only exacerbated with long-haul, international flights. With larger planes with greater numbers of passengers, and potentially hundreds of people in the aircraft cabin breathing and rebreathing the same air, ventilation becomes critical to eliminate possible contaminants and airborne infections and provide environmental comfort. In modern aircrafts, 50% of fresh air is introduced and added to 50% of recirculated air. While this is an improvement when compared to ventilation averages for public and commercial buildings, which combine 20% of fresh air with 80% of recirculated air, the population density is much higher in aircraft compared to most commercial buildings and public spaces [23].

On long-haul international flights, travelers spend longer periods in enclosed spaces, especially those which can facilitate the spread of infectious diseases. Several outbreaks of serious infectious diseases have been reported aboard commercial airlines since 1946, including influenza, measles, severe acute respiratory syndrome (SARS), tuberculosis, food poisoning, viral enteritis, and small pox [3].

Most commercial aircraft use high-efficiency particulate air filters to recirculate the cabin air. There appears to be little or no difference between types of air filters used: one study showed no significant difference in self-reported infection rates in aircraft that use high-efficiency particulate air filters compared with those in aircraft that use a single-pass cabin ventilation system [24].

The risk of onboard transmission of infection is mainly restricted to individuals either with close personal contact or seated within two rows of an index passenger [25, 26]. However, in one report of a single flight on Air China flight 112, 22 passengers and crew member developed probable onboard severe acute respiratory syndrome-associated coronavirus (SARS-CoV) infection [27].

According to the World Health Organization (WHO) and multiple other studies, the 2002–03 SARS epidemic indicated that commercial air travel has an effect on infectious-disease spread [28]. WHO estimates that "65 passengers per million who travelled aboard commercial flights originating from regions of active transmission during the outbreak were symptomatic with probable SARS" [28]. WHO estimates that during the SARS epidemic, 40 flights carried 37 probable SARS-CoV source cases during the outbreak, resulting in 29 probable onboard secondary cases [28].

It is likely, based upon data from these and other studies, as well as from the contained environment and prolonged exposure to rebreathed and recycled air, that these international flights pose a significant exposure risk to various infectious diseases.

4.5 Vector- and Insect-Borne Diseases on International Flights

As far back as 1933, it was recognized that air travel posed a risk for insect-borne diseases:

The first sanitary convention for aerial navigation was conducted in 1933 and recognized the importance of aviation to the worldwide community. One of the focused concerns was control of the yellow fever mosquito vector. Following World War II, the WHO Committee on Hygiene and Sanitation in Aviation became activated and published the "Guides to Hygiene and Sanitation in Aviation." The most recent guide is dated 1977 [23].

In the last 50 years, insects and other vectors for malaria, dengue, and yellow fever have all been identified on aircraft. Further, a condition termed "airport malaria" refers to cases of malaria near international airports among people who have not recently traveled into endemic areas. In the past 30, years most European countries, the United States, Israel, and Australia have experienced confirmed or probable cases of airport malaria. In the last 30 years, the United States has reported four such cases [23].

Both the WHO and the Advisory Group for Aerospace Research and Development recommend "aircraft disinsection" given evidence that disease vectors, particularly mosquitoes, are being imported into countries on aircraft [29].

4.6   Risk of Deep Venous Thromboembolism in International Travelers

Some members of the traveling public have a genetic tendency for increased clotting that has been estimated to have a prevalence of as high as 20% in the general population. Other preexisting factors such as illness, smoking, and medication may represent preexisting risk factors leading to deep venous thrombosis (DVT) during or following traveling [23].

Until recently, reviews of the medical literature failed to find significant epidemiological studies that demonstrate a statistically significant increase in DVT as a result of traveling by any means in the absence of preexisting risk factors. In the absence of any good prospective published studies, the evidence linking DVT with flying is likely circumstantial [30].

However, according to Silverman 2008, the relationship between long-haul flights (>8 h) and increased risk of DVT has generated great interest in both medical publications and the media. Overall, studies show an association between venous thromboembolism and long-haul air travel, with risk up to fourfold, depending on study methods [31–37]. In their review article in *The Lancet* in 2008, Silverman et al. provided an overview of the mildly increased risk of DVT associated with air travel [3].

In 2001, the Air Transport Medicine Committee of the Aerospace Medical Association recommended that "passengers with no identifiable risk factors carry out frequent and regular stretching exercises particularly of the lower limbs during flight. Opportunities should be sought to change position in the seat as well as to walk about the cabin. For those with more identifiable risk factors it is recommended that the traveler seek advice from his or her personal physician" [30].

Silverman and colleagues describe risks of venous thromboembolism (VTE), consolidating various recommendations in the literature [3]. For example, for low-risk passengers on short-duration flights, passengers are encouraged to avoid constrictive clothing and dehydration while also ambulating about the cabin when possible, whereas high-risk passengers on longer flights are potential candidates for low-molecular-weight heparin [3, 31–37]. Generally, there is high risk for VTE only in flights of more than 8 h [38] and the risk of VTE usually occurs only in flights of more than 4 h [6, 33].

4.7 Special Medical Equipment Needs for International Flights

Several resources are available to providers who respond to a medical emergency. The Federal Aviation administration (FAA) mandates that United States-based airlines carry first-aid kits that are stocked with basic supplies such as bandages and splints [39].

These supplies are not comprehensive (e.g., there are no pediatric or obstetrical supplies). An Aerospace Medical Association expert panel has recently recommended an expanded cache [40].

Because health professionals are not aboard every flight, most airlines contract with ground-based medical consultation services [41, 42]. The clinicians at these centers can provide treatment recommendations. Onboard volunteer providers can also consult these services during an emergency. In demanding situations that require more than one provider, a volunteer physician may ask whether other medical professionals can assist [38]. The FAA also mandates that flight attendants receive training every other year in cardiopulmonary resuscitation (CPR) and the use of AEDs [17, 42, 43].

4.8 Emergency Medical Kits on International Flights

The first emergency medical kit was mandated by the FAA in 1986 and was subsequently expanded in 2001 to include an inhaled bronchodilator, oral antihistamines, and nonnarcotic analgesics [44]. Beginning in 2004, the FAA required all commercial airlines with at least a 7,500-lb payload and one or more flight attendants to equip their planes with AEDs [44]. The emergency medical kit is intended for use by medically-trained professionals responding to an emergency onboard an aircraft and includes the items listed in Table 1.1. The medical kits that can be found on international airlines are different from those found on US carriers and usually represent an expanded version of the US kit.

According to Kahn et al. [44] and DeJohn et al. [45], several studies have been conducted, analyzing the usefulness of the FAA-mandated emergency medical kit:

> A survey of health care professionals who had used the kit to manage emergencies aboard aircraft found that whereas 26% thought it was "very useful," 55% found it only "somewhat useful," and 18% believed that the kit was "not of any benefit." [45]

A study by De John et al. [45] of 1,132 in-flight medical incidents on 5 US domestic airlines found that the emergency medical kit was opened 47% of the time overall and 65% of the time when a flight was diverted. In addition to the items included in the kit, healthcare professionals believed that the following were also very helpful a majority of the time when managing medical emergencies: supplemental oxygen, supportive care, and careful patient monitoring [44, 45].

4.9 Special Areas for Critical Patients on International Flights

Several airlines provide specialized sections and/or small rooms on board their international flights. Lufthansa has developed a patient-transport compartment (PTC) for intensive care on board Lufthansa commercial long-distance aircraft on intercontinental routes. The configuration consists of a small enclosed room placed in the middle row of wide-body international aircraft. Three rows of seats are removed to make room for the PTC. Backup devices are present for all vital medical equipment (for monitoring, artificial ventilation, infusions, etc.) in case of failure. Thirteen thousand liters of oxygen (gas volume) are carried on the flight. The patient is accompanied by one intensive care nurse and one physician [2]. Other airlines describe modifications of this concept, allowing a special, isolated space for critical patients requiring ongoing medical monitoring and care, rather than for providing space to treat in-flight medical emergencies; however, if present and unoccupied by other patients, these spaces could be used for in-flight emergency patients [2].

4.10 Legal Issues

Liability: An issue of concern to many healthcare professionals when deciding whether to volunteer assistance in a medical emergency onboard a plane is the legal liability issues involved. A physician who provides assistance creates a doctor–patient relationship, with its attendant obligations and liability risk. Most doctors are eager to help in an emergency but are concerned that doing so might put them at risk; however, there have been numerous "Good Samaritan" laws enacted to protect healthcare professionals who respond in emergency situations. In 1998, Congress enacted the US Aviation Medical Assistance Act, which outlines protection for physicians and airlines who provide emergency medical care for passengers on commercial airliners, provided that the physician acts in good faith, receive no monetary compensation, provide reasonable care, and does not "grossly neglect" the patient or commit "willful misconduct." An example of such disregard would be an intoxicated physician treating a patient [46]. Furthermore, many airlines indemnify volunteering physicians, and the captain should provide written confirmation on request [3, 11]. In addition, the insurance policies of many airlines cover healthcare professionals who provide emergency medical care to passengers or crew while on board their aircraft [46].

The situation is a bit more complicated for medical professionals traveling on an international flight, however, as he or she becomes subject to the laws of the country in which the airline is registered. These laws may differ significantly from those of the United States. New Zealand, for example, requires that medically qualified persons respond to a medical emergency, and failure to do so is grounds for legal action [46, 47].

According to British, Canadian, and US laws, medical professionals are not required to volunteer assistance during an in-flight medical event, unless they have a preexisting clinical relationship with the passenger. In contrast, physicians in Australia and many Asian, European, and Middle Eastern countries are required to provide assistance [41]. For international flights, the country where the aircraft is registered has jurisdiction, except when the aircraft is on the ground or in sovereign airspace [11, 41]. Medical assistance during an in-flight medical event is typically protected under Good Samaritan laws [3, 8, 48].

Documentation: According to the recommendations made by the International Air Transport Association (IATA), in-flight medical emergencies should be documented properly for a variety of reasons [42]. A recent study reported preliminary evidence that the documentation of in-flight medical emergencies is not as consistent as one would expect. Of the 32 European airlines that were asked to contribute data on in-flight medical emergencies, only 4 airlines were able to potentially provide the necessary data [14].

After the event, the provider should document the care that was provided and the treatment that was delivered and should use airline-specific documentation as required [42]. Providers should be mindful of the patient's privacy rights and should not discuss the patient's care with third parties (e.g., media) without appropriate authorization from the patient [49]. The captain of the aircraft and the flight crew should receive appropriate medical information to support correct medical management and allow for appropriate flight diversion. The airline itself is not obligated to follow federal regulations regarding healthcare privacy, because it is not considered to be a covered entity [17, 47].

In general, there is a large variation in the documentation of in-flight medical emergencies between airlines, and a higher degree of standardization is preferable for medical care, for research, and to meet the IATA recommendations [47].

4.11 Future Recommendations

Registries of in-flight emergencies: The lack of an international registry with valid data and sound denominator data impedes quality research in this area. To date, neither a national nor a European/international standardized registry on in-flight medical emergencies exists. Presently, only company registers of specific airlines are available toward this end [10]. The lack of a central registry makes it difficult to conduct research as to the true incidence of in-flight events [10, 14]. The information gained from epidemiologic studies of in-flight medical emergencies is of benefit to the airlines, aerospace medical researchers, and the traveling public [5, 50, 51].

Training of airline personnel: In-flight medical emergencies occur frequently, and available evidence suggests that there is significant room to improve and standardize the care that is provided to patients during in-flight medical emergencies.

The US Federal Aviation Administration (FAA) mandates that flight attendants receive training "to include performance drills, in the proper use of AEDs and in CPR [cardiopulmonary resuscitation] at least once every 24 months" [52, 53]. However, the FAA "does not require a standard curriculum or standard testing" [52, 53].

Many airlines also contract with a commercial on-ground support company that can, in theory, offer radioed, real-time medical advice. To improve the chances that passengers who become ill during air travel will do well, airlines and their regulators could take steps similar to what they have done to ensure flight safety for all flights under FAA jurisdiction [52–54].

Other improvements for the future: The following suggestions are made from multiple studies examining long-haul in-flight emergencies:

1. A standardized recording system for all in-flight medical emergencies should be adopted, with mandatory reporting of each incident to the National Transportation Safety Board, the organization responsible for reviewing safety events and recommending changes to practice.
   (a) A survey of European airlines identified 10,000 in-flight medical emergencies during a 5-year period [13]. The study noted that each airline had its own reporting system and protocol.
2. The optimal content of first aid kits on airplanes should be determined, with a mandate that a standard kit, with identical elements, in identical locations, be on every flight [13].
   (a) Even though emergency medical kits are mandated to contain certain medications and equipment, the actual kits vary from airline to airline [52, 53].
3. The training of flight attendants in how to deal with medical emergencies should be enhanced and standardized.
   (a) The US Federal Aviation Administration (FAA) mandates that flight attendants receive training "to include performance drills, in the proper use of AEDs] and in CPR [cardiopulmonary resuscitation] at least once every 24 months" [52, 53]. However, the FAA "does not require a standard curriculum or standard testing" [52, 53].
4. Access of flight crews to ground-to-air medical support should be standardized.
   (a) Many airlines also contract with a commercial on-ground support company that can, in theory, offer radioed, real-time medical advice [54].

References

1. Rodenberg H. Medical emergencies aboard commercial aircraft. Ann Emerg Med. 1987;16:1373–7.
2. Graf J, Stüben U, Pump S. In-flight medical emergencies. Dtsch Arztebl Int. 2012;109:591–601; quiz 602.
3. Silverman D, Gendreau M. Medical issues associated with commercial flights. Lancet. 2008;373:2067–77.
4. Peterson DC, Martin-Gill C, Guyette FX, et al. Outcomes of medical emergencies on commercial airline flights. N Engl J Med. 2013;368:2075–83.
5. Hinkelbein J, Neuhaus C, Böhm L, Kalina S, Braunecker S. In-flight medical emergencies during airline operations: a survey of physicians on the incidence, nature, and available medical equipment. Open Access Emerg Med. 2017;9:31–5.
6. Kesapli M, Akyol C, Gungor F, Janitzky Akyol A, Soydam Guven D, Kaya G. Inflight emergencies during Eurasian flights. J Travel Med. 2015;22(6):361–7.
7. Qureshi A, Porter KM. Emergencies in the air. Emerg Med J. 2005;22:658–9.
8. Bourell L, Turner M. Management of in-flight medical emergencies. J Oral Maxillofac Surg. 2010;68:1377–83.
9. Jagoda A, Pietrzak M. Medical emergencies in commercial air travel. Emerg Med Clin North Am. 1997;15:251.
10. Ruskin K. In-flight medical emergencies: time for a registry? Crit Care. 2009;13:121.
11. Cocks R, Liew M. Commercial aviation, in-flight emergencies and the physician. Emerg Med Australas. 2007;19:1–8.
12. Cummins RO, Schubach JA. Frequency and types of medical emergencies among commercial air travelers. JAMA. 1989;261:1295–9.
13. Sand M, Bechara FG, Sand D, Mann B. In-flight medical emergencies. Lancet. 2009;374:1062–3.
14. Sand M, Bechara FG, Sand D, Mann B. Surgical and medical emergencies on board European aircraft: a retrospective study of 10189 cases. Crit Care. 2009;13(1):R3.
15. Delaune EF III, Lucas RH, Illig P. In-flight medical events and aircraft diversions: one airline's experience. Aviat Space Environ Med. 2003;74:62.
16. Garrett JS. Twelve thousand inflight medical emergencies: what have we learned? Air Med J. 2000;19:110.
17. Nable J, Tupe C, Gehle B, Brady W. In-flight medical emergencies during commercial travel. N Engl J Med. 2015;373:939–45.
18. Dowdall N. 'Is there a doctor on the aircraft?' Top 10 in-flight medical emergencies. BMJ. 2000;321:1336–7.
19. Select Committee on Science and Technology. Air travel and health: fifth report. London: House of Lords; 2000.
20. Shepherd B, Macpherson D, Edwards CMB. In-flight emergencies: playing The Good Samaritan. J R Soc Med. 2006;99:628–31.
21. Derlet R, Richards J. In-flight emergencies at 35,000 feet. Cal J Emerg Med. 2005;6(1):14–8.
22. Valani R, Cornacchia MK, Ube D. Flight diversions due to onboard medical emergencies on an international commercial airline. Aviat Space Environ Med. 2010;81:1037–40.
23. DeHart R. Health issue of air travel. Annu Rev Public Health. 2003;24:133–51.
24. Zitter JN, Mazonson PD, Miller DP, Hulley SB, Balmes JR. Aircraft cabin air recirculation and symptoms of the common cold. JAMA. 2002;288:483–6.
25. Mangili A, Gendreau MA. Transmission of infectious diseases during commercial air travel. Lancet. 2005;365:989–96.
26. WHO. Tuberculosis and air travel: guidelines for prevention and control. WHO/HTM/TB/2006.363. 2nd ed. Geneva: World Health Organization; 2006.
27. Olsen SJ, Chang HL, Cheung TY, et al. Transmission of the severe acute respiratory syndrome on aircraft. N Engl J Med. 2003;349:2416–22.

28. WHO. Department of communicable disease surveillance and response. Consensus document on the epidemiology of severe respiratory distress syndrome (SARS). WHO/CDS/CSR/2003.11. Geneva: World Health Organization; 2003.

29. Gratz NG, Steffen R, Cocksedge W. Why aircraft disinsection? Bull WHO. 2000;78:997–1013.

30. Bagshaw M. Travellers' thrombosis: a review of deep vein thrombosis associated with travel. The Air Transport Medicine Committee, Aerospace Medical Association. Aviat Space Environ Med. 2001;72:848–51.

31. Arya R, Barnes JA, Hossain U, Patel RK, Cohen AT. Long-haul flights and deep vein thrombosis: a significant risk only when additional factors are also present. Br J Haematol. 2002;116:653–4.

32. Becker NG, Salim A, Kelman CW. Air travel and the risk of deep vein thrombosis. Aust NZ J Public Health. 2006;30:5–9.

33. Cannegieter SC, Doggen CJ, van Houwelingen HC, Rosendaal FR. Travel-related venous thrombosis: results from a large population-based case control study (MEGA study). PLoS Med. 2006;3:e307.

34. Ferrari E, Chevallier T, Chapelier A, Baudouy M. Travel as a risk factor for venous thromboembolic disease: a case-control study. Chest. 1999;115:440–4.

35. Gallus AS. Travel, venous thromboembolism, and thrombophilia. Semin Thromb Hemost. 2005;31:90–6.

36. Kuipers S, Cannegieter SC, Middeldorp S, Robyn L, Buller HR, Rosendaal FR. The absolute risk of venous thrombosis after air travel: a cohort study of 8,755 employees of international organisations. PLoS Med. 2007;4:e290.

37. Martinelli I, Taioli E, Battaglioli T, et al. Risk of venous thromboembolism after air travel: interaction with thrombophilia and oral contraceptives. Arch Intern Med. 2003;163:2771–4.

38. Baltsezak S. Clinic in the air? A retrospective study of medical emergency calls from a major international airline. J Travel Med. 2008;15:391–4.

39. Federal Aviation Administration (FAA), Department of Transportation. Emergency medical equipment: final rule. Fed Regist. 2001;66:19028–46.

40. Aerospace Medical Association, Air Transport Medicine Committee. Medical emergencies: managing in-flight medical events. Virginia: Aerospace Medical Association; 2013.

41. Gendreau MA, DeJohn C. Responding to medical events during commercial airline flights. N Engl J Med. 2002;346:1067–73.

42. International Air Transport Association. Medical manual. 7th ed. Montreal: IATA; 2006. Goodwin T. In-flight medical emergencies: an overview. BMJ 2000; 321: 1338-41.

43. Federal Aviation Administration (FAA). Advisory circular: emergency medical equipment training. AC No. 121-34B. Washington, DC: Federal Aviation Administration; 2006. http://www.faa.gov/documentLibrary/media/Advisory_Circular/AC121-34B.pdf

44. Kahn RA, Ruckman RF, Brown SB, et al. Case 3-2006 Cardiac arrest at 30,000 feet. J Cardiothorac Vasc Anesth. 2006;20:438.

45. DeJohn CA, Veronneau SJH, Wolbrink AM, et al. An evaluation of the U.S. in-flight medical kit. Aviat Space Environ Med. 2002;73:496.

46. Aviation Medical Assistance Act of 1998, Pub L. No. 105–170, vol. 1998. Washington, DC: National Archives and Records Administration.

47. Sand M, Morrosch S, Sand D, Altmeyer P, Bechara F. Medical emergencies on board commercial airlines: is documentation as expected? Crit Care. 2012;16:R42, 2-7.

48. Kuczkowski K. "Code blue" in the air: implications of rendering care during in-flight medical emergencies. Can J Anaesth. 2007;54(5):401–2.

49. Health Insurance Portability and Accountability Act of 1996 (HIPAA), Pub. L. No. 104–191, 110 Stat. 1936. Washington, DC: National Archives and Records Administration, 1996.

50. Hinkelbein J. Significant more research required: no further progress without sound medical data and valid denominators for in-flight medical emergencies. J Travel Med. 2015;22(6):355–6.

51. Hinkelbein J, Spelten O, Wetsch WA, et al. Emergencies in the sky: in-flight medical emergencies during commercial air transport. Trends Anaesth Critical Care. 2013;3:179–82.

52. US Federal Aviation Administration. Emergency medical equipment: advisory circular 121-
    33B. http://rgl.faa.gov/Regulatory_and_Guidance_Library/rgAdvisoryCircular.nsf/key/AC%20
    121-33B!OpenDocument. Accessed 8 May 2017.
53. US Federal Aviation Administration. Emergency medical equipment training: advisory circu-
    lar 121-34B. http://www.faa.gov/regulations_policies/advisory_circulars/index.cfm/go/docu-
    ment.information/documentID/22519. Accessed 8 May 2017.
54. Mattison M, Zeidel M. Navigating the challenges of in-flight emergencies. JAMA.
    2011;305(19):2003–4.

In-Flight Evaluation and Management of Cardiac Illness

5

François-Xavier Duchateau, Tobias Gauss,
Matthew Beardmore, and Laurent Verner[†]

5.1 Introduction

Cardiac diseases represent the most frequent in-flight emergencies (almost 50% of cases) and the overwhelming majority of diversions (81.3%), according to a recent study of 11,920 in-flight emergency calls from 5 airlines to a physician-directed medical communications center over 2 years [1]. In addition to their frequency, the acute presentation of cardiac diseases may result in a poor outcome, with some situations requiring immediate emergency treatment [2]. This chapter provides epidemiological information, an approach to risk stratification of patients when considering the need to divert the aircraft, and a suggested guide on how to handle in-flight cardiac emergencies, including cardiac arrest, acute myocardial infarction, and decompensated congestive heart failure.

5.2 Cardiac Arrest

In-flight cardiac arrest occupies a very specific place among in-flight emergencies since it requires specific skills and the ability to perform CPR in a very unaccommodating environment; it also represents a very significant challenge for those with little or no practical experience of such situations—this situation would also

[†]Deceased

F.-X. Duchateau, M.D. (✉) • L. Verner, M.D.
Allianz Worldwide Partners, Group Medical Direction, Saint Ouen, France
e-mail: francois-xavier.duchateau@allianz.com

T. Gauss, M.D.
HEMS, East Anglian Air Ambulance, Norwich, UK
e-mail: tobias.gauss@aphp.fr

M. Beardmore, M.B., Ch.B. (Hons)
Department of Anesthesiology, Peninsula Deanery, Plymouth, UK
e-mail: mdbeardmore@doctors.org.uk

© Springer International Publishing AG, part of Springer Nature 2018
J. V. Nable, W. Brady (eds.), *In-Flight Medical Emergencies*,
https://doi.org/10.1007/978-3-319-74234-2_5

challenge the seasoned clinician. This condition is fortunately quite rare, representing only 0.3% of in-flight emergencies, but is responsible for 86% of in-flight events resulting in death [1]. The rate of survival after cardiac arrest on commercial aircrafts improved dramatically after the introduction of automated external defibrillators (AED) on board. It ranges from 14 to 55%, with the best outcomes for patients presenting with witnessed collapse and ventricular fibrillation (VF) [3, 4]. Programs combining the installation of automatic external defibrillator (AED) devices aboard aircraft with training of the cabin crew in extrication of unconscious passengers from their seat, cardiopulmonary resuscitation (CPR), and use of AEDs were demonstrated to have a positive impact on survival [3].

The airline cabin presents a challenging environment for resuscitation. It is very confined with limited ability to move around the patient and perform appropriate interventions. Unless the help of a second CPR-capable healthcare professional is available, a basic compression-only approach is recommended. Diversion should be promptly considered and the aircraft captain informed and updated throughout the resuscitation attempt. Potential reasons for non-diversion include the following: diversion is not feasible (e.g., while the aircraft is crossing the ocean); when the airplane is close to the scheduled destination; and diversion does not offer any advantages compared to continuing on the scheduled route.

Proposed guide for the management of in-flight cardiac arrest:

- Recognize cardiac arrest.
- Request for AED to be brought urgently to patient.
- Request for extrication of the patient from his/her seat to the nearest available space by the crew: ideally the galley or a door bay.
- Expose patient's chest.
- If AED is available, apply pads and connect to device; perform AED rhythm analysis and shock if applicable, and then start compressions (compression-only CPR).
- If AED is not available or shock unsuccessful, start compression-only CPR, which offers the best balance of practicality and efficacy [5, 6]; conventional CPR with chest compressions and bag-valve mask ventilation can be considered if a second CPR-capable healthcare professional is present [7]; compression-only CPR, however, is appropriate with several available rescuers.

If return of spontaneous circulation (ROSC) is achieved, post-resuscitation measures remain basic. While not evidence-based, administering oxygen is one of the few available supportive measures that might be of benefit. Essentially, the role of the medical volunteer will be to monitor the patient until appropriate ground-based resources take over the patient's management. Diversion to the nearest appropriate location is mandatory; the patient's condition remains critical and the medical volunteer needs to advise the aircraft captain to divert immediately. The AED should remain connected and ready for any further life-threatening arrhythmias.

The International Air Transport Association requires that the emergency medical kit contain 1 mg epinephrine vials, allowing the provision of more advanced life support by medical volunteers capable of such measures [8]. In the case of non-shockable rhythms, the insertion of an IV line and administration of 1 mg epinephrine may be considered.

Where resuscitation efforts are unsuccessful, particularly in the presence of a non-shockable rhythm, it is reasonable to cease all efforts after 20–30 min. The very poor anticipated outcome, even with appropriate basic resuscitation in this austere environment, makes the prolonged continuation of efforts futile if the patient does not respond quickly to such measures [9]. In the circumstance of shock-resistant/refractory VF/VT cardiac arrest, with the AED continuing to deliver shocks, resuscitation efforts should be continued until the ground-based resources take care of the patient [7], assuming that diversion and emergency landing are possible within a very short period of time; in this situation, if emergency landing cannot occur rapidly due to reasons beyond the control of the medical personnel, and the patient remains in cardiac arrest with a shockable rhythm, prolonged resuscitation is unlikely to result in a good outcome—thus, resuscitation efforts can be stopped after approximately 30 min of resuscitation.

Only a physician has the authority to pronounce death aboard an aircraft. In this case, the captain may reasonably challenge the value of diverting since there is no longer any therapeutic benefit in doing so, although the emotional impact on any relatives present as well as the other passengers will have to be factored into this decision.

5.3   Acute Myocardial Infarction

Based on the findings of the previously cited study, "cardiac symptoms," among which chest pain is at the forefront, represent 8% of in-flight emergencies [1]. Other common presentations such as syncope or pre-syncope (37% of in-flight medical emergencies), "respiratory symptoms" (12%), and cardiac arrest (0.3%) may be related to underlying coronary disease and acute coronary syndrome. None of the current major airlines are equipped with telemetry devices that would provide a 12-lead electrocardiogram (ECG) and thus guide the appropriately trained clinician in the evaluation of the patient; this type of equipment, however, does exist in the innovation phase of development. Without an ECG, acute myocardial infarction (AMI) will be only suspected based on patient's history and a brief, focused physical examination. Because exacerbation of preexisting conditions represents 65% of in-flight emergencies and the large majority of de novo medical presentations are with syncope [10], eliciting a past medical history of coronary disease is of value in the assessment.

The medical challenge here is determining the probability of an acute coronary syndrome without the help of the ECG or cardiac biomarkers. Few scoring systems have been developed and assessed within these particular constraints and we suggest a basic, qualitative approach. Identified predictive factors of AMI or unstable angina are older age (greater than 40 years); a history of exertional angina; typical angina pain as the main complaint; hypotension; and acute heart failure [11, 12].

Typically, ischemic cardiac pain is characterized by a sensation of squeezing, heaviness, pressure, weight, vicelike aching, burning, or tightness in the chest with radiation to shoulder, neck, jaw, inner arm, or epigastrium (the latter features may occur without chest discomfort) [13]. The most significant and sensitive physical findings include pale appearance, diaphoresis, and anxiety.

Several important considerations must be addressed in the patient with chest pain or other complaints, reflective of acute coronary syndrome. In cases of likely acute coronary syndrome, in an ill-appearing patient or in patients presenting with unstable features, the captain should be advised to divert immediately.

Conversely, for a stable patient who is at low risk for an acute coronary syndrome, it seems reasonable to continue to the scheduled destination, assuming that arrival is anticipated within several hours; furthermore, arrangements should be made for patient transfer to a facility capable of evaluation upon landing. Between these two ends of the spectrum, the patient should receive the benefit of the doubt and diversion should be advised.

Therapeutic measures are limited in flight. In the absence of active, clinically significant bleeding or true allergic reaction, aspirin (160–324 mg) is recommended in adult patients with chest pain who are suspected of having an acute coronary syndrome [14]. There is no indication for P2Y12 inhibitors or anticoagulation, without formal investigations to confirm the diagnosis, since the risk-benefit balance is uncertain and the patient will be exposed to an increased risk of hemorrhage. Furthermore, it is unlikely that these agents will be available. While IATA regulations mandate their presence in the standardized medical kit of commercial airliners, nitroglycerin tablets are of uncertain therapeutic benefit while potentially resulting in severe side effects such as hypotension or even being harmful in cases of inferior AMI with right ventricular involvement. Their use without the ability to more fully assess and monitor the patient should be done so with caution. Even when there is no apparent respiratory compromise, supplemental oxygen will improve oxygenation since commercial airliners are usually pressurized to the regulatory maximum equivalent altitude of 8,000 ft. [15]. In cases where AMI is strongly suspected, applying AED pads and having the AED ready for the potential development of ventricular fibrillation would be prudent.

5.4   Syncope

Syncope and pre-syncope are the most frequent conditions (37–52%) occurring aboard commercial flights, according to the most recent large cohort studies [3, 16]. From a pathophysiological perspective, there are many reasons for passengers to present with faintness, pre-syncope, and syncope aboard commercial airliners, especially during long-haul flights. Because airliners are pressurized to the equivalent altitude of 6,000–8,000 ft., resulting in a lower partial pressure of oxygen, passengers experience a relative hypoxia at cruising altitude. Cabin pressurization is achieved by pumping non-humidified air through the engines and, despite recirculating humidified air from the cabin, this results in a relatively arid environment.

Altered eating patterns, consumption of alcohol, use of sedation agents, fatigue, and sleep deprivation may also contribute [2]. Each of these individual factors alone could be the cause of syncope or pre-syncope but the presence of multiple contributing factors makes this presentation very common. Besides these causes related to the environment, more serious conditions such as pulmonary embolism and arrhythmia should be considered, particularly if the patient does not quickly return to baseline, if the patient has significant past medical history suggestive of past similar events related to serious pathology, and/or if the history of the present episode suggests severe event etiology.

The onset of this clinical presentation can be both impressive and alarming to all passengers involved. The medical volunteer needs to carefully assess the situation and act immediately when indicated. Initial assessment should include assessment of consciousness, pulse, and blood pressure; if still unconscious, the simple maneuver of elevating the legs with the patient lying down on the floor may provide relief. While the device may not be universally present in the cabin medical kit, where possible, the blood glucose level should be checked with a finger prick device [2] and any demonstrated hypoglycemia corrected, using available resources and considering the patient's mental status and ability (or inability) to safely take oral carbohydrate.

For patient with persistent hypotension despite the above measures, intravenous (IV) line insertion and normal saline fluid loading are potentially indicated. For patients with persistent bradycardia, the administration of IV atropine may be considered by medical personnel familiar with its use; the risk:benefit balance must be considered in each case, with clinical features such as extreme bradycardia or pauses favoring carefully titrated administration [17].

In the case of rapid resolution of symptoms in a previously healthy person, it is reasonable to advise against diversion and continue to the flight's scheduled destination, assuming that the patient has returned to baseline health state, is symptom-free, has no significant preexisting conditions, and is assessed to be at low risk of developing new medical problems. Identification of a trigger factor for syncope is a plus. The patient should be advised to seek medical advice upon arrival.

Conversely, persistent symptoms, significant preexisting conditions, or presence of very significant cardiac risk factors are independent arguments in favor of a recommendation to divert and request ground-based resources be present on landing.

5.5   Congestive Heart Failure

The nature of in-flight epidemiological data, subclassifying patients into having pulmonary compromise and/or respiratory distress, limits the ability to understand the prevalence of congestive cardiac failure in this setting. It would not be sound to be more specific and distinguish pulmonary edema from exacerbations of a lung disease, indeed nor from other acute respiratory diseases. Respiratory symptoms represent 12% of in-flight emergencies [1]. A proportion of these emergencies are related to acute cardiac failure. Of particular note, pulmonary hypoxemia and alcohol intake may have a role in the development of congestive cardiac failure [18].

Correctly diagnosing acute decompensated heart failure is a clinical challenge for physicians regardless of setting [18] and we expect that this challenge is even more difficult aboard an aircraft since chest auscultation is impaired by the noise of the engines. A history of previous heart failure has the best predictive value in the diagnosis. Symptoms of worsening fluid retention or decreasing exercise tolerance related to increasing left or right ventricular filling pressures are often present. Potential precipitants such as ischemia, medication noncompliance, dietary indiscretions, arrhythmias, and hypertension are other potential features favoring the diagnosis. Inquire about the presence of chest pain and other features of acute coronary syndromes given that acute cardiac failure may be the mode of presentation of an AMI.

The principal measure is the administration of supplemental oxygen. The patient should remain in the sitting position. Furosemide is included in the standard medical kit as recommended by the International Air Transport Association and may be of particular interest in patients with clinical features of fluid overload when available [18]. Nitroglycerin tablets can help by lowering afterload, and thus left-sided filling pressures, and may be administered, especially in the presence of systemic hypertension (and contraindicated if systolic blood pressure is less than 100 mmHg).

Diversion for ground-based rescue should be advised in most suspected cases of decompensated heart failure as therapeutic options on board are very limited. It may be reasonable to continue to the scheduled destination only when the patient's symptoms are very mild, anticipated time to scheduled landing is relatively short, and/or the available ground-based resources are insufficient.

References

1. Peterson DC, Martin-Gill C, Guyette FX, et al. Outcomes of medical emergencies on commercial airline flights. N Engl J Med. 2013;368:2075–83.
2. Nable JV, Tupe CL, Gehle BD, Brady WJ. In-flight medical emergencies during commercial travel. N Engl J Med. 2015;373:939–45.
3. O'Rourke MF, Donaldson E, Geddes JS. An airline cardiac arrest program. Circulation. 1997;96:2849–53.
4. Brown AM, Rittenberger JC, Ammon CM, Harrington S, Guyette FX. In-flight automated external defibrillator use and consultation patterns. Prehosp Emerg Care. 2010;14:235–9.
5. Rea TD, Fahrenbruch C, Culley L, et al. CPR with chest compression alone or with rescue breathing. N Engl J Med. 2010;363:423–33.
6. Svensson L, Bohm K, Castrèn M, et al. Compression-only CPR or standard CPR in out-of-hospital cardiac arrest. N Engl J Med. 2010;363:434–42.
7. Kleinman ME, Brennan EE, Goldberger ZD, et al. 2015 American Heart Association Guidelines Update for Cardiopulmonary Resuscitation and Emergency Cardiovascular Care. Part 5: Adult Basic Life Support and Cradiopulmonary Resuscitation Quality. Circulation. 2015;132:S414–35.
8. IATA. Guidance on managing medical events. 2015. https://www.iata.org/whatwedo/safety/Documents/IATA-Guidance-on-Managing-Medical-Events.pdf. Accessed 26 Feb 2017.
9. Mancini ME, Diekema DS, Hoadley TA, et al. 2015 American Heart Association Guidelines Update for Cardiopulmonary Resuscitation and Emergency Cardiovascular Care. Part 3: ethical issues. Circulation. 2015;132:S383–96.

10. Qureshi A, Porter KM. Emergencies in the air. Emerg Med J. 2005;22:658–9.
11. Geleijnse ML, Elhendy A, Kasprzak JD, et al. Safety and prognostic value of early dobutamine-atropine stress echocardiography in patients with spontaneous chest pain and a non-diagnostic electrocardiogram. Eur Heart J. 2000;21:397–406.
12. Pollack CV Jr, Braunwald E. 2007 update to the ACC/AHA guidelines for the management of patients with unstable angina and non-ST-segment elevation myocardial infarction: implications for emergency department practice. Ann Emerg Med. 2008;51:591–606.
13. Sangareddi V, Chockalingam A, Gnanavelu G, Subramaniam T, Jagannathan V, Elangovan S. Canadian Cardiovascular Society classification of effort angina: an angiographic correlation. Coron Artery Dis. 2004;15:111–4.
14. AHA Part 10.
15. Aerospace Medical Association, Aviation Safety Committee, Civil Aviation Subcommittee. Cabin cruising altitudes for regular transport aircraft. Aviat Space Environ Med. 2008;79:433–9.
16. Sand M, Bechara FG, Sand D, et al. Surgical and medical emergencies on board European aircraft: a retrospective study of 10,189 cases. Crit Care. 2009;13:R3.
17. Link MS, Berkow LC, Kudenchuk PJ, et al. 2015 American Heart Association Guidelines Update for Cardiopulmonary Resuscitation and Emergency Cardiovascular Care. Part 7: Adult Advanced Cardiovascular Life Support. Circulation. 2015;132:S444–64.
18. Kapoor JR, Perazella MA. Diagnostic and therapeutic approach to acute decompensated heart failure. Am J Med. 2007;120:121–7.

Respiratory Emergencies

6

Kami M. Hu

6.1 Introduction and Epidemiology

Respiratory illnesses are some of the most common in-flight complaints, accounting for up to 14% [1, 2] of the medical emergencies that occur on commercial flights. Spontaneous or de novo respiratory emergencies can and do occur, but in-flight respiratory complaints are more often due to exacerbations of existing pulmonary disease, including chronic obstructive pulmonary disease (COPD) and pulmonary hypertension. In 2015, there were 36.5 million smokers in the United States, with 40% having smoking-related lung disease [3]. Anywhere from 18 to 44% of air travelers carry a diagnosis of COPD, and approximately 25% of flyers with COPD experience symptoms of hypoxia in-flight [4]. As the obesity crisis continues, conditions that predispose to the development of secondary pulmonary hypertension, such as obstructive sleep apnea and obesity hypoventilation syndrome, are on the rise [5]. The aging of the US population also contributes to a higher number of patients with a diagnosis of either primary or secondary pulmonary hypertension, patients who also develop symptomatic hypoxia in the air [6]. A wide range of patients are at-risk of decompensation at altitude, including those with cystic lung diseases, those who have had recent thoracic surgery or trauma, and even those with primary cardiac disease presenting as respiratory distress. Healthcare providers responding to these in-flight complaints should be familiar with altitude-related physiologic changes that may play a role in the patient's presentation, as well as the management options available to them in the air.

K. M. Hu, M.D.
Departments of Emergency Medicine and Internal Medicine,
University of Maryland School of Medicine, Baltimore, MD, USA
e-mail: khu@som.umaryland.edu

© Springer International Publishing AG, part of Springer Nature 2018
J. V. Nable, W. Brady (eds.), *In-Flight Medical Emergencies*,
https://doi.org/10.1007/978-3-319-74234-2_6

6.2   Respiratory Physiology While Flying

Simply *being* on a commercial flight results in relative hypoxemia and can cause physiologic stress to the patient with or without chronic respiratory illness. Standard cruising altitudes for most modern commercial aircraft are anywhere from 22,000 to 48,000 [7]; while the Federal Aviation Administration (FAA) mandates that the aircraft cabin be pressurized to no higher than 8,000 ft, pressures consistent with higher altitudes have been documented in up to 10% of flights [8]. At these higher altitudes, the atmospheric and partial pressures of oxygen are lower, resulting in relative hypoxemia in even the healthiest flying patient, with an arterial oxygen partial pressure (PaO_2) of approximately 60 millimeters of mercury (mmHg), as opposed to 100 mmHg at sea level.

This concept is explained by Dalton's law of partial pressures, which states that the total pressure of a gas—in this instance, atmospheric pressure—is equivalent to the sum of the partial pressures of all the gases that comprise it. Atmospheric pressure at sea level is 760 mmHg, but at higher altitudes the atmospheric pressure is lower, as less of the atmosphere is above to "weigh it down." The atmospheric pressure at an altitude of 40,000 ft is 140 mmHg, but, by pressurizing the cabin, the atmospheric pressure is brought up to approximately 590 mmHg. As the atmospheric pressure decreases, so too do the individual partial pressures of each gas. While the percentage of oxygen in the air remains a stable 21%, the partial pressure of oxygen—both in the cabin and in patient circulation—is lower at cruising altitude than at sea level. Another way to understand the decrease in inspired oxygen is to look at the equation for inspired oxygen tension (PiO_2):

$$PiO_2 = FiO_2 \times \left(P_{atm} - PH_2O \right)$$

As the plane ascends and atmospheric pressure decreases, PiO_2, and therefore the alveolar partial pressure of oxygen (PAO_2) will also decrease, resulting in a decreased gradient from alveoli to the arterial circulation, and a decreased PaO_2.

This hypobaric hypoxic state is usually well tolerated by healthy travelers, as they remain on the normoxemic area of the oxygen-dissociation curve (Fig. 2.1). Patients who start with a lower PaO_2 at sea level end lower on the curve, making it harder for the oxygen to dissociate from hemoglobin in order to be available for use by the tissues, and leading to symptoms indicative of a hypoxemic state (Fig. 2.1).

The increase in altitude has the additional effect of gas expansion, which can cause pneumothorax, pneumomediastinum, systemic air embolism secondary to cyst or bleb rupture, or can worsen existing pneumothoraces. This gas expansion is explained by Boyle's law, which states that in a closed system, for instance the airplane or a cystic lung lesion, at a constant temperature, the volume of a gas is inversely proportional to its pressure. As the gas pressure decreases at cruising altitude, there is a resultant 25–30% gas expansion within enclosed spaces [9]. This expansion affects not only bullae in the lungs but all closed systems on the aircraft, including the sinuses, gastrointestinal tract, and medical devices, such as feeding tube and urinary catheter balloons.

6.3   Preparing for Air Travel

The best way to manage hypoxic events in flight is to prevent them with proper pre-flight preparation. Patients with chronic lung diseases should be evaluated by their primary physician and/or pulmonologist to determine their fitness for air travel. Historically, three main methods have been described to predict fitness to fly and the need for in-flight oxygen: the 50-meter (m) walk test, equations utilizing sea level measurements of pulmonary function, and hypoxia challenge testing (HCT). HCT, also called hypoxia altitude simulation testing (HAST), is the current gold standard assessment for predicting supplemental oxygen need in flight [10–12]. This test simulates the hypoxic environment of cruising altitude either by using an actual hypobaric chamber or by having patients breathe a fraction of inspired oxygen (FiO_2) of 15% mixed with nitrogen gas for 20 minutes (min) before assessing their peripheral oxygen saturation (SpO_2) and PaO_2 by arterial blood gas. In patients without usual need for supplemental oxygen, a $PaO_2 \leq 50$ mmHg or $SpO_2 \leq 85\%$ on HCT is an indication for 2 L/min of oxygen during air travel [13].

While its simplicity is attractive, there is no data to support the use of the 50-m walk test. In fact, one study found that an inability to walk 330 meters, rather than 50, was the functional finding that correlated to hypoxic results on HCT [14]. The assumption that the ability to walk 50 meters affirms fitness to fly without oxygen is therefore faulty, and would inevitably send people on flights to become hypoxic, perhaps with great detriment to their health. Unfortunately, the different predictive equations that have been developed to estimate the predicted PaO_2 at altitude are also flawed [14, 15]. These equations incorporate various measurements made at sea level, such as the forced expiratory volume in 1 second (FEV_1), forced vital capacity (FVC), diffusion capacity (DLCO), SpO_2, and PaO_2. Several of these measures, namely FEV_1 and DLCO, do seem to correlate with hypobaric oxygen levels [14] but there has not yet been any validation of an equation including them. While undoubtedly less involved than HCT, existing predictive equations are inaccurate with poor reproducibility and are not recommended.

How then should physicians determine whom to refer for official hypoxic challenge testing? The most widely published guidelines, those from the British Thoracic Society (BTS), recommend formal hypoxic challenge testing for patients with an SpO_2 of 92–95% and any of the following: hypercapnia, $FEV_1 < 30\%$ predicted, lung cancer, restrictive lung disease (including those involving chest wall or respiratory muscle disease), ventilator support, cerebrovascular or cardiac disease, or within six weeks of discharge for an exacerbation of chronic lung or cardiac disease [13]. The different recommendations from the variety of major societies on respiratory or aviation medicine are listed in Table 6.1 [12, 13, 16–19].

For passengers who may not fall into one of these categories, a noninvasive yet reliable method to determine a need for supplemental oxygen versus additional testing is to monitor SpO_2 before and during the standard 6-minute walk test [20] (Table 6.2). Validated in COPD patients, a need for in-flight oxygen is indicated if the patient's resting SpO_2 is less than 92% at rest or if it falls below 84% during exertion. Patients will not require oxygen if their resting SpO_2 is greater than 95%

Table 6.1 Patient factors requiring further evaluation for supplemental oxygen need [12, 13, 16–19]

Organization(s)	Factors
British Thoracic Society [13]	SpO$_2$ 92–95% AND one of the following: – Hypercapnia – FEV$_1$ < 30% predicted – Lung cancer – Restrictive lung disease – Ventilator support – Cerebrovascular/cardiac disease – Flight within 6 weeks from exacerbation of chronic lung or cardiac disease
American Thoracic Society [16] European Respiratory Society [16]	Any of the following: – COPD with comorbidities – Prior history of in-flight symptoms – Recent exacerbation of pulmonary disease – Hypoventilation with oxygen administration
Aerospace Medical Association [17] Canadian Thoracic Society [18]	PaO$_2$ < 70 mmHg at sea level
Department of Veterans Affairs [19]	COPD with frank or borderline hypoxia (SpO$_2$ < 90%)

SpO$_2$ peripheral oxygen saturation, *PaO$_2$* arterial partial pressure of oxygen, *COPD* chronic obstructive pulmonary disease, *mmHg* millimeters of mercury

Table 6.2 Interpretation of the 6-minute walk test [20]

	Resting SpO$_2$		
6MWT SpO$_2$	<92%	92–95%	>95%
<84%	In-flight O$_2$	In-flight O$_2$	Proceed to HCT
≥84%	In-flight O$_2$	Proceed to HCT	No O$_2$ needed

6MWT 6-minute walk test, *SpO$_2$* percent oxygen saturation

and remains 84% or greater during exertion. Patients who fall between these two categories, who have a resting SpO$_2$ between 92 and 95% without desaturation to less than 84%, or who have a resting SpO$_2$ > 95% but desaturate, should be referred for HCT, as these values did not consistently and accurately predict in-flight hypoxemia in the validation study [20]. Of note, there is small-study data to indicate that a baseline SpO$_2$ > 95% does not rule out a need for in-flight oxygen in severe asthmatics, and therefore all severe asthmatics should undergo HCT prior to air travel [21].

It is important for patients who are already dependent on supplemental oxygen to know that the FAA does not allow patients to fly with their own oxygen tanks, but some airlines will provide oxygen to travelers with prior notification (how far in advance depends upon the airline) and an additional fee. The number of these airlines has decreased however; the majority of domestic US airlines do not provide oxygen beyond emergency situations, choosing to recommend portable oxygen concentrators (POCs) instead. All airlines with flights originating or ending in the United States are required to allow the use of a POC, although it must be one of the FAA-approved machines [22] (Table 6.3). Patients dependent on supplemental

Table 6.3 Portable oxygen concentrators approved by the Federal Aviation Administration for use in flight [22]

Company	Model(s)
AirSep	Focus, FreeStyle, FreeStyle 5, LifeStyle
Caire	Model 4000
Delphi Medical Systems	RS-00400
DeVilbiss Healthcare	IGo (306DS)
Inogen	One, One G2, One G3
Inova Labs/International Biophysics	LifeChoice, LifeChoice Activox
Invacare	XPO2, Solo2 (TPOC)
Oxlife	Independence
Oxus	RS-00400
Precision Medical	EasyPulse (PM4150)
Respironics	EverGo, SimplyGo (E2)
SeQual	Eclipse, eQuinox, Oxywell, SAROS (3000)
VBox	Trooper

oxygen at sea level should expect to have their oxygen requirement increase by 1–2 LPM [16]; the BTS guidelines recommend doubling the flow rate in flight [13], but these patients may also undergo HCT in order to determine what their in-flight requirement will be. The maximum oxygen deliverable by most POCs and commercial aircraft is approximately 3 and 4 LPM, respectively; therefore an oxygen requirement greater than 3-4 LPM at sea level may preclude travel by air [16].

6.4 Preflight Recommendations by Disease Process

General rules of thumb for patients with lung disease who plan to travel include evaluation by their primary doctor/pulmonologist/specialist prior to flight, inclusion of medications and therapeutic devices in carry-on luggage with extra supplies (batteries, infusion pumps/tubing, etc.), and advance notification of the airline if any accommodations are needed. More specific advice varies depending on the illness; some recommendations by disease process are included below.

6.4.1 Obstructive Airway Disease (Asthma, COPD)

For patients with mild to moderately severe asthma, flights rarely cause problems other than the minor exacerbation improved with inhaled bronchodilator usage [13]. Smoking-related lung disease is, of course, somewhat different from asthma in terms of its physical and physiologic effects on the human body. Patients with emphysema or COPD may have preexisting hypoventilation, a lower baseline arterial oxygen tension, ventilation-perfusion mismatch, and/or bullae that put them at risk for pneumothorax at altitude. Despite these points, the frequency of severe adverse events reported in this population actually remains fairly low [4, 14].

Patients with severe asthma should consult with their pulmonologist and optimize their therapy prior to air travel. All patients with obstructive lung disease should keep their pulmonary medications, including an emergency steroid, in their carry-on luggage.

6.4.2   Pneumothorax/Recent Thoracic Surgery

Current recommendations on how soon to fly after pneumothorax resolution are varied. The Aerospace Medical Association (AsMA) recommends a delay of 14–21 days after resolution of a pneumothorax [17], while the BTS and International Air Transport Association (IATA) recommend a delay of 7 days after thoracic surgery or resolution of spontaneous pneumothorax, and a delay of 14 days after traumatic pneumothorax, in addition to a chest X-ray that confirms resolution prior to flight. Although there little reliable data to make strict guidelines, the general consensus is that patients with active pneumothorax without a chest tube and release valve should not fly. Of note, there are case reports of patients with chronic, loculated pneumothorax flying without complication [23, 24].

Patients with cystic lung diseases have long been thought to be at increased risk of in-flight pneumothorax due to the expansion of gases at higher altitudes. With the exception of lymphangioleiomyomatosis (LAM), a rare disease causing cystic lung destruction that carries documented increased risk of spontaneous pneumothorax at sea level, there is no data to support that concern. Physicians should warn patients of the potential risk of pneumothorax prior to air travel, but there are no particular precautions to be taken.

6.4.3   Obstructive Sleep Apnea (OSA)

Patients planning to sleep in flight should bring their continuous positive airway pressure (CPAP) machine in their carry-on. Prior to their flight, they should check with the company that manufactured their device to ensure that it will work in the low-pressure cabin environment. They should also have dry-cell batteries, as A/C power is often not readily available in the cabin. These patients should also avoid alcohol and sedatives before and during travel, as these can worsen respiratory depression by increasing apnea durations and exacerbating air-exchange difficulties while napping in flight [25, 26].

6.4.4   Pulmonary Arterial Hypertension (PAH)

Hypobaric hypoxia can worsen pulmonary hypertension by inducing pulmonary vasculature vasoconstriction [27]; patients with PAH must be evaluated by their pulmonologist or pulmonary hypertension specialist prior to flight for HCT referral. The Pulmonary Hypertension Association recommends that patients who use epoprostenol travel with a small cooler holding extra medicine, including a pre-mixed dose, and that patients who use continuous infusion pumps carry an extra pump with them [28].

6.4.5 Interstitial Lung Disease

These patients should be evaluated by their pulmonologists prior to air travel to evaluate the need for HCT, if not already on supplemental oxygen. Additionally, they may need to carry antibiotics for use if needed, and have an emergency steroid or escalated-dose regimen available if they are already on chronic steroid therapy.

6.4.6 Heart Failure

Patients with even relatively severe stable heart failure without significant pulmonary hypertension generally do well with the mild hypoxia of air travel [29, 30]. The BTS recommends HCT in heart failure patients who are hypoxemic at sea level and have coexisting lung disease, but states that otherwise patients in stable New York Heart Association (NYHA) functional classes I–III can fly without supplemental oxygen. Patients with NYHA class IV symptoms are advised not to fly, but, if they must, to fly with supplemental oxygen of at least 2 LPM [13].

6.5 In-Flight Emergency Management

When a respiratory emergency occurs in flight, the options for intervention are limited. The initial evaluation and management of travelers presenting with shortness of breath or an increased work of breathing should follow these general steps:

– *Check vital signs and administer supplemental oxygen.* Portable pulse oximeters are not mandated by the FAA for inclusion in the emergency medical kits (EMK) carried on board; however some airlines carry additional medical supplies in addition to the basic kit. It is reasonable to have the flight attendant check if one is present and/or survey the other passengers via the overhead announcement system to see if one is available. A search for pulse oximeter should not delay administration of supplemental oxygen.
– *Listen for lung sounds and assess patient for tracheal deviation.* The initial goal is to discover a tension pneumothorax, if present, as it could be rapidly fatal if missed. Unfortunately, auscultation onboard an airplane may be of low yield, but, if audible, the presence of adventitious lung sounds can guide further management steps.
– *Consider requesting the pilot descend to lower altitude, if appropriate, and contact ground medical consultant, if available.* Although not required by the FAA, many airlines contract with a local hospital or medical consulting team that can

be reached at any time. These medical consultants are usually much more familiar with the physiologic effects of cruising altitude on the body, the contents of the airline's emergency medical kit, and options for intervention in-flight. They can assist in deciding whether or not the flight should be diverted, although it should be noted that the final decision regarding diversion rests with the captain.

More specific management of patients with dyspnea will depend, of course, on their full clinical picture. Acute respiratory distress with the presence of crackles should prompt further evaluation to determine possible etiology: Are there signs of volume overload? Is the patient severely hypertensive? In patients with mild or even slightly moderate symptoms, application of supplemental oxygen, perhaps also with a single dose of nitroglycerin, can be enough to temporize them until the flight destination is reached. Nitroglycerin is provided in all FAA-mandated EMKs, and can be administered for patients with acute decompensated heart failure or acute hypertensive pulmonary edema. Some airline emergency kits also carry a diuretic, which can be administered if the patient is having moderate-to-severe symptoms. It is important to keep in mind that the patient may not be able to make repeated trips to the lavatory, whether due to symptoms or flight turbulence. If prompt fluid removal is necessary, a substitute urinal should be provided. Some airlines' medical kits also include an additional medication that can lower blood pressure, such as a beta-blocker, the use of which emergency responders can consider on a case-by-case basis. Routine use of longer acting blood pressure medications is not recommended, as there are limited means to raise the blood pressure if the effect is too strong.

Dyspnea with the presence of wheezes should receive bronchodilator by metered-dose inhaler (MDI); if the patient has a personal inhaler, that inhaler should be used preferentially. If the clinical picture does not completely improve or the patient is exhibiting moderate-to-severe respiratory distress, it is reasonable to see if there is an MDI spacer onboard the flight, as administration of bronchodilator via an MDI with spacer is equivalent to administration using a nebulizer [31, 32]. Some passengers will carry a nebulizer onboard or travel with a smaller portable nebulizer. These can be used in flight, although the oxygen flow rates supplied by the airplane may be limited. Sharing of nebulizers between passengers is not recommended due to concerns regarding communicable disease. Providers should consider intramuscular or subcutaneous epinephrine 1:1,000 (0.3–0.5 milligrams, mg) for patients with severe respiratory distress secondary to asthma. Epinephrine is not advised for patients with exacerbations of COPD, who often have concomitant cardiac dysfunction as well as much less airway disease reversibility than patients with asthma, and therefore confers a smaller benefit. If the EMK contains a corticosteroid, whether oral or injectable, administer a single dose.

If there is concern for dyspnea secondary to allergic reaction, bronchodilator by MDI should be administered; intramuscular (IM) epinephrine 1:1,000 should be considered early and should absolutely be given at the first sign of anaphylaxis (0.2–0.5 mg IM or subcutaneously every 5 min as needed). These patients should receive diphenhydramine 10–50 mg IM or IV every 2–3 hours (h), although oral diphenhydramine can be given if the patient is not in severe respiratory distress or in danger of losing his or her airway, 25–50 mg every 4–6 h as needed (maximum diphenhydramine dose is 400 mg in a day). Administration of a corticosteroid, if present in the kit, may help decrease the occurrence of biphasic anaphylaxis, although there is no conclusive data to this effect [33]. A patient requiring administration of epinephrine for anaphylaxis should prompt consideration for aircraft diversion, especially if the dose must be repeated. Any allergic reaction that causes real potential for loss of the airway due to airway edema should also prompt serious consideration for diversion of the aircraft.

If diversion is not a possibility (i.e., the aircraft is flying over the ocean) and/or airway loss is impending, the responding provider should consider proceeding with cricothyrotomy, depending on their level of training and specialty. Rationale for earlier initiation of this procedure invokes the consideration that it is easier to perform a task in a relatively controlled setting rather than while the patient is crashing and has no other way to breathe. "Quick-cric" kits exist but are not likely to be found onboard during a flight; improvisation in this setting is key. Cleaning of the area should be undertaken with soap and water, isopropyl alcohol, alcohol-based hand sanitizer, or even the highest proof liquor available. Lidocaine can be obtained from the EMK and administered locally prior to incision with scissors, pocketknife, or other sharp objects sterilized with alcohol and a lighter or match. Endotracheal tubes are not provided in the basic EMKs, and improvisation with plastic straws from water bottles, cutoff syringes without the stoppers, an IV tubing drip chamber and spike, and even ballpoint pens (with an internal lumen greater than 4 mm) have been documented as successful [34–37] and should be considered. Without an endotracheal tube and its connector, connecting the makeshift airway to the BVM can be difficult. A method using the nipple from a infant's bottle has also been described [37].

If the patient's dyspnea corresponds with clinical evidence of a tension pneumothorax, the patient should be immediately placed on supplemental oxygen and consideration for descent to a lower altitude should be discussed with the flight crew. This reverses the expansion of gas within the pleural cavity to decrease the volume of the pneumothorax and strain on the heart. The immediate next step is to perform a needle thoracostomy (NT). Classic teaching is that the preferred NT site is the second intercostal space in the midclavicular line, most commonly using a standard 14-gauge IV-start needle at least 5 centimeters (cm) in length. Several studies have demonstrated, however, that many patients have a greater chest wall diameter that prevents successful breach of the pleural cavity with this method [36, 37]. Of note, the FAA mandates neither specific NT devices nor 5-cm 14-gauge needles for inclusion in the aircraft EMKs. For these reasons, unless the patient is thin, it is more appropriate to attempt thoracostomy at the fourth or fifth intercostal space in the anterior axillary line using the longest available needle available, with larger gauge being a secondary consideration. The needle should be inserted just above the rib bone to avoid injuring the neurovascular bundle that runs along the underside of each separate rib. Providers should strongly consider using an IV-start needle if one of the appropriate lengths is available, as it can be stabilized with tape against the chest wall, with the catheter in the pleural space and the hub connected to a syringe to prevent re-accumulation, as a means for repeated decompression if needed. Alternately, the catheter can be inserted through a disposable glove (although a sterile glove would be more ideal) into the chest wall, and the freely hanging glove over the hub can serve as a flap valve. It is important to note that the catheter may kink or dislodge at any time—the patient should remain closely monitored, and a contingency plan is important.

Whether or not the NT is successful, the responder should take inventory of items that could be possibly used to perform more invasive thoracostomy. If the NT is not successful and the patient is decompensating, the next immediate step for the trained physician should be a finger thoracostomy [38, 39]. Additional cleaning of the area should be undertaken with available disinfectants as mentioned above and lidocaine should be administered subcutaneously for local anesthesia. A scalpel is clearly preferred for the procedure, but the scissors from the EMK or another sharp knife or razor, sterilized with alcohol and a lighter, may be the only available option. As the ribs and intercostal muscle are reached, the closed scissors can be used to poke through the muscle (again, just above the rib to avoid neurovascular injury) and then the index finger used to make the full breach. In this manner, a pneumothorax can be diagnostically verified and treated simultaneously even if there are no supplies to perform a chest tube insertion [40, 41]. It should be noted that a makeshift chest tube has been successfully fashioned and inserted on a commercial flight using scissors, a wire hanger, a urinary catheter, a bottle of water, tape, oxygen tubing, and brandy [42].

In the case of hypoventilatory respiratory failure, respiratory support can readily be offered via the use of a bag-valve-mask. An oropharyngeal airway can and should be used only if the patient's gag reflex is not intact. Hypercapnia should be considered in passengers presenting with depressed mental status who are at risk for obstructive sleep apnea or obesity hypoventilation syndrome, and is managed by bagging the patient with good mask seal, timed with their respirations, giving additional breaths if needed. A slow respiratory rate should evoke the possibility of opiate-induced hypoventilation and trigger the administration of naloxone, if available. Naloxone is not included in all EMKs; however due to recent pushes by nationwide health departments to make it available to all members of the public, it is reasonable to ask overhead if any other passengers are carrying it.

Conclusion

Respiratory illnesses remain one of the more common complaints that arise during commercial flights, a trend not likely to change as the population ages and the obesity epidemic continues. Fortunately, respiratory events at cruising altitude do not often result in severe adverse outcomes. Unfortunately, when the respiratory distress is severe, the available interventions are limited. The true preparation for in-flight respiratory emergencies mainly lies in prevention—namely, ensuring that patients who would go on to become dangerously hypoxic in flight are identified prior to travel in order to access supplemental oxygen. The remaining preparation lies in the motivation of healthcare providers to familiarize themselves with the physiologic effects of flying, the tools they will have on board, and the improvisations they may need to use to save a life 40,000 ft in the air.

References

1. Peterson DC, Martin-Gill C, Guvett FX, Tobias AZ, McCarthy CE, Harrington ST, et al. Outcomes of medical emergencies on commercial airline flights. N Engl J Med. 2013;368(22):2075–83.
2. Chandra A, Conry S. In-flight medical emergencies. West J Emerg Med. 2013;14(5):499–504.
3. Centers for Disease Control and Prevention. Cigarette smoking among adults—United States, 2005–2015. Morb Mortal Wkly Rep. 2016;65(44):1205–11.
4. Edvardsen A, Akerø A, Hardie JA, Ryg M, Eagan TM, Skjønsberg OH, Bakke PS. High prevalence of respiratory symptoms during air travel in patients with COPD. Respir Med. 2011;105(1):50–6.
5. Balachandran JS, Masa JF, Mokhlesi B. Obesity hypoventilation syndrome epidemiology and diagnosis. Sleep Med Clin. 2014;9(3):341–7.
6. Roubinian N, Elliott CG, Barnett CF, Blanc PD, Chen J, De Marco T, Chen H. Effects of commercial air travel on patients with pulmonary hypertension. Chest. 2012;142(4):885–92.
7. Mohr LC. Hypoxia during air travel in adults with pulmonary disease. Am J Med Sci. 2008;335(1):71–9.
8. Hampson NB, Kregenow DA, Mahoney AM, et al. Altitude exposures during commercial flight: a reappraisal. Aviat Space Environ Med. 2013;84(1):27–31.
9. Silverman D, Gendreau M. Medical issues associated with commercial flights. Lancet. 2009;373(9680):2067–77.
10. Kelly PT, Swanney MP, Seccombe LM, Frampton C, Peters MJ, Beckert L. Air travel hypoxemia vs. the hypoxia inhalation test in passengers with COPD. Chest. 2008;133:920–6.
11. Dine CJ, Kreider ME. Hypoxia altitude simulation test. Chest. 2008;133(4):1002–5.
12. Akero A, Edvardsen A, Christensen CC, Owe JO, Ryg M, Skjønsberg OH. COPD and air travel: oxygen equipment and preflight titration of supplemental oxygen. Chest. 2011;140(1):84–90.
13. Ahmedzai S, Balfour-Lynn IM, Bewick T, Buchdahl R, Coker RK, Cummin AR, et al. Managing passengers with stable respiratory disease planning air travel: British Thoracic Society recommendations. Thorax. 2011;66:i1–i30.
14. Bradi AC, Faughnan ME, Stanbrook MB, Deschenes-Leek E, Chapman KR. Predicting the need for supplemental oxygen during airline flight in patients with chronic pulmonary disease: a comparison of predictive equations and altitude simulation. Can Respir J. 2009;16(4):119–24.
15. Martin SE, Bradley JM, Buick JB, Bradbury I, Elborn JS. Flight assessment in patients with respiratory disease: hypoxic challenge testing vs. predictive equations. QJM. 2007;100(6):361–7.
16. Celli BR, Decramer M, Wedzicha JA, Wilson KC, Agusti A, Criner GJ, et al. ATS/ERS Task Force for COPD Research. An official American Thoracic Society/European Respiratory Society Statement: research questions in chronic obstructive pulmonary disease. Am J Respir Crit Care Med. 2015;191(7):e4–e27.
17. Medical guidelines for airline travel, 2nd ed. Aviat Space Environ Med. 2003;74(5 Suppl):A1–19.
18. Lien D, Turner M. Recommendations for patients with chronic respiratory disease considering air travel: a statement from the Canadian Thoracic Society. Can Respir J. 1998;5(2):95–100.
19. The Management of Chronic Obstructive Pulmonary Disease Working Group. VA/DoD clinical practice guideline for the management of chronic obstructive pulmonary disease. 2014. http://www.healthquality.va.gov/guidelines/CD/copd/VADoDCOPDCPG2014.pdf. Accessed 19 Jan 2017.
20. Edvardson A, Akero A, Christensen CC, Rvg M, Skjønsberg OH. Air travel and chronic obstructive pulmonary disease: a new algorithm for pre-flight evaluation. Thorax. 2012;67(11):964–9.

21. George PM, Orton C, Ward S, Menzies-Gow A, Hull JH. Hypoxic challenge testing for fitness to fly with severe asthma. Aerosp Med Hum Perform. 2016;87(6):571–4.
22. Federal Aviation Association: Regulatory and guidance library. 2016. http://rgl.faa.gov. Accessed 19 Jan 2017.
23. Currie GP, Kennedy AM, Paterson E, Watt SJ. A chronic pneumothorax and fitness to fly. Thorax. 2007;62(2):187–9.
24. Hu X, Cowl CT, Bagir M, Ryu JH. Air travel and pneumothorax. Chest. 2014;145(4):688–94.
25. Mitler MM, Dawson A, Henriksen SJ, Sobers M, Bloom FE. Bedtime ethanol increases resistance of upper airways and produces sleep apneas in asymptomatic snorers. Alcohol Clin Exp Res. 1988;12(6):801–5.
26. Roehrs T, Roth T. Sleep, sleepiness, sleep disorders and alcohol use and abuse. Sleep Med Rev. 2001;5(4):287–97.
27. Turner BE, Hodkinson PD, Timperley AC, Smith TG. Pulmonary artery pressure response to simulated air travel in a hypobaric chamber. Aerosp Med Hum Perform. 2015;86(6):529–34.
28. The Pulmonary Hypertension Association. Traveling with PH. 2017. http://phassociation.org/Patients/TravelingWithPH#air. Accessed 19 Jan 2017.
29. Smith D, Toff W, Joy M, Dowdall N, Johnston R, Clark L, et al. Fitness to fly for passengers with cardiovascular disease. Heart. 2010;96(Suppl 2):ii1–16.
30. Ingle L, Hobkirk J, Damy T, Nabb S, Clark AL, Cleland JG. Experiences of air travel in patients with chronic heart failure. Int J Cardiol. 2012;158(1):66–70.
31. Newman KB, Milne S, Hamilton C, Hall K. A comparison of albuterol administered by metered-dose inhaler and spacer with albuterol by nebulizer in adults presenting to an urban emergency department with acute asthma. Chest. 2002;121(4):1036–41.
32. Cates CJ, Welsh EJ, Rowe BH. Holding chambers (spacers) versus nebulisers for beta-agonist treatment of acute asthma. Cochrane Database Syst Rev. 2013;9:CD000052.
33. Lieberman P, Nicklas RA, Oppenheimer J, Kemp SF, Lang DM, Bernstein DI, et al. The diagnosis and management of anaphylaxis practice parameter: 2010 update. J Allergy Clin Immunol. 2010;126(3):477–80.
34. Braun V, Kisser U, Huber A, Stelter K. Bystander cricothryoidotomy with household devices—a fresh cadaveric feasibility study. Resuscitation. 2017;110:37–41.
35. Platts-Mills TF, Lewin MR, Wells J, Bickler P. Improvised cricothyrotomy provides reliable airway access in an unembalmed human cadaver model. Wilderness Environ Med. 2006;17(2):81–6.
36. Owens D, Greenwood B, Galley A, Tomkinson A, Woolley S. Airflow efficacy of ballpoint pen tubes: a consideration for use in bystander cricothyrotomy. Emerg Med J. 2010;27(4):317–20.
37. Iserson KV. Airway. In: Iserson KV, editor. Improvised medicine: providing care in extreme environments. 2nd ed. New York, NY: McGraw-Hill; 2016. http://accessemergencymedicine.mhmedical.com/content.aspx?bookid=1728&Sectionid=115694410. Accessed 10 Jan 2017.
38. Inaba K, Branco BC, Eckstein M, Shatz DV, Martin MJ, Green DJ, et al. Optimal positioning for emergent needle thoracostomy: a cadaver-based study. J Trauma. 2011;71(5):1099–103.
39. Inaba K, Ives C, McClure K, Branco BC, Eckstein M, Shatz D, et al. Radiologic evaluation of alternative sites for needle decompression of tension pneumothorax. Arch Surg. 2012;147(9):813–8.
40. Fitzgerald M, Mackenzie CF, Marasco S, Hoyle R, Kossman T. Pleural decompression and drainage during trauma reception and resuscitation. Injury. 2008;39(1):9–20.
41. Massarutti D, Trillo G, Berlot G, Tomasini A, Bacer B, D'Orlando L, et al. Simple thoracostomy in prehospital trauma management is safe and effective: a 2-year experience by helicopter emergency medical crews. Eur J Emerg Med. 2006;13(5):276–80.
42. Wallace TW, Wong T, O'Bichere A, Ellis BW. Managing in flight emergencies. BMJ. 1995;311(7001):374–6.

Neurological Illness

7

Sara A. Hefton and Wan-Tsu W. Chang

7.1   Epidemiology

Neurological emergencies are one of the most common in-flight medical emergencies during commercial travel. They account for up to 30% of all in-flight medical consultations [1, 2]. Neurological cases are also the second most common cause of diversions [1]. As the general population ages and commercial travel continues to increase, the incidence of neurological complaints during flights will likely increase. It is important for the clinicians who may be called upon to care for these patients during flight to be able to identify critical neurological conditions that require time-sensitive interventions and potential diversion.

While in-flight neurological emergencies are common, only 12% require diversion [1]. This may be due to a subset of events that are related to preexisting medical conditions or minor symptoms triggered by the stress of air travel. Diversion is more common with loss of consciousness, altered mental status, stroke-like symptoms, and seizures [2]. A clinician needs to be able to distinguish the acuity and urgency of in-flight neurological complaints in order to provide advice to the flight staff and ground medical consultation on the recommended management. A clinician also needs to be able to manage these events utilizing limited equipment available on the aircraft and resources provided by flight staff and ground medical consultation.

S. A. Hefton, M.D.
Department of Neurological Surgery, Division of Neuro-Trauma and Critical Care,
Thomas Jefferson University, Philadelphia, PA, USA
e-mail: sara.hefton@jefferson.edu

W.-T. W. Chang, M.D. (✉)
Department of Emergency Medicine, University of Maryland School of Medicine,
Baltimore, MD, USA
e-mail: wchang@em.umaryland.edu

© Springer International Publishing AG, part of Springer Nature 2018   65
J. V. Nable, W. Brady (eds.), *In-Flight Medical Emergencies*,
https://doi.org/10.1007/978-3-319-74234-2_7

7.1.1 Stroke

Stroke symptoms account for 2% of in-flight medical emergencies. However, it is the most common reason for hospital admission [3]. Air travel increases the risk of stroke due to multiple factors. The partially pressurized cabins result in a lower ambient partial oxygen pressure and can increase the risk of ischemic stroke in patients without adequate cerebrovascular reserve. The low humidity in the cabin air can contribute to dehydration, thereby increasing the risk of thrombotic events such as cerebral venous thrombosis [4]. In addition, restricted mobility can result in venous thrombosis of the legs and paradoxical embolization in patients with a right-to-left shunt [5, 6].

A survey of pilots using simulated in-flight scenarios found that pilots were less likely to use ground medical consultation and to declare an emergency for stroke than for myocardial infarction. Pilots were also less likely to respond for younger patients and posterior circulation stroke symptoms than for elderly patients and anterior circulation stroke symptoms. One out of five pilots that participated in this study did not think that stroke could be treated [7]. These findings suggest that education of pilots is an important aspect of managing in-flight stroke symptoms.

7.1.2 Seizure

Seizures and postictal states comprise 5.8% of in-flight medical emergencies [3]. Seizure threshold is lowered by air travel due to hypoxemia and disruption of the passengers' circadian rhythms. In addition, alcohol consumption can also lower seizure threshold. In a review of in-flight medical consultations over a 6-year period, seizures had a similar likelihood of diversion as stroke symptoms. Factors that contributed to the diversion were status epilepticus, repetitive seizures with intermittently preserved consciousness, prolonged postictal states, injury, and febrile convulsions in infants [2].

7.1.3 Altered Mental Status

Altered mental status represents a significant portion of in-flight medical emergencies. The causes of altered mental status may be neurologic, metabolic, infectious, toxicological, or psychiatric in origin. The true incidence of in-flight altered mental status emergencies is unclear, as the lack of standardized categorizations has led to flight and medical consultation records grouping these emergencies into "confusion," "unresponsiveness," "other neurologic," "diabetic complication," etc. [2, 3, 8]. One retrospective study found that patients who were reported to be unconscious were 33 times more likely to require diversion and 234 times more likely to die during flight [9]. However, it is unclear what were the underlying etiologies of these patients' unconscious states.

Given the broad differential diagnoses and the limited diagnostic capabilities on an aircraft, a detailed history and physical are important to help narrow the potential etiologies in order to determine necessary interventions, some of which may be time-sensitive. Persistently altered mental status raises concerns about conditions such as stroke that should prompt consideration of diversion.

7.1.4   Dizziness

Dizziness is the most common in-flight neurological emergency reported. It is also the most common neurological symptom resulting in diversion [2]. The etiology of dizziness is broad, spanning neurological conditions such as vertebrobasilar insufficiency, cardiopulmonary conditions such as arrhythmias or hypoxia, and otological conditions such as Ménière's disease. In addition, changes in cabin pressure can cause passengers to experience symptoms of acute mountain sickness [10].

7.1.5   Headache

Headache is an infrequently reported in-flight medical emergency. Of all neurological cases, it is likely the most underestimated. Cabin pressure changes, disruptions of circadian rhythms, consumption of alcohol, and stress of air travel can all contribute to headaches. However, many occurrences are likely self-treated. Passengers who request medical assistance with their headaches are, in essence, self-selected from benign causes and should be treated with a high index of suspicion.

7.1.6   Head Injury

Head injury is the second most common type of traumatic injury in flight. These injuries often result from blunt trauma due to turbulence. Although many are not serious, clinicians should consider risk factors for traumatic intracranial hemorrhage such as age and anticoagulant use. Frequent reassessment of the patient will also allow for observation of the patient's status and recognition of any worsening that should signal an intracranial injury needing escalation of care.

7.2   Risk Stratification

In general, approach to in-flight neurological emergencies begins with a thorough history and neurological examination given the limited diagnostic capabilities on an aircraft. The clinician should obtain details regarding time of onset, progression of symptoms, associated symptoms, as well as whether the patient has had similar symptoms previously. In the case of stroke-like symptoms, details regarding the time of onset would help the clinician determine whether the patient may be a candidate for reperfusion therapy and coordinate the logistics of potential diversion with the flight staff and ground medical consultation. For patients with severe headaches, a history of sudden-onset worst headache of life may be concerning for a subarachnoid hemorrhage and thus increase the urgency in definitive medical treatment.

A detailed neurological examination is helpful in risk-stratifying patients with in-flight neurological symptoms. A new neurological deficit is worrisome for an acute neurological emergency and warrants urgent medical evaluation. Acute-onset unilateral weakness or speech deficit is concerning for stroke, and similar symptoms associated with altered mental status are concerning for intracranial hemorrhage, both needing diversion for time-sensitive treatment. Hypoglycemia and infections can exacerbate existing neurological deficits from an old stroke. However, the absence of neurological deficits does not preclude a neurological emergency. Stroke-like symptoms that have resolved at the time of evaluation by the clinician are concerning for a transient ischemic attack (TIA). While patients with TIA symptoms are at higher risk of subsequent stroke and would benefit from urgent medical evaluation, the decision to recommend diversion to the flight crew would likely need to be made on a case-by-case basis considering associated risks and benefits. Patients with subarachnoid hemorrhage may only complain of worst headache of life but otherwise be neurologically intact and still have a high risk of neurological deterioration from rebleeding, hydrocephalus, and seizures. Head injury of significant mechanism may be concerning for an epidural hematoma even if the patient became "lucid" after an initial loss of consciousness. Thus, perhaps more important than a detailed neurological examination is a repeated neurological assessment to evaluate the progression of symptoms and better determine the urgency of definitive medical evaluation.

Lastly, a complete physical examination and evaluation of the surroundings are also important, as in-flight neurological symptoms such as altered mental status may be a sequelae of a medical condition. Findings of alcohol or medications may increase the suspicion of intoxication or overdose. An arteriovenous fistula or a tunneled dialysis catheter would add electrolyte derangements and uremia to the differential diagnoses. Fever, rash, or an obvious wound would heighten the suspicion for an infection. While medical illnesses with associated neurological complications may not require diversion, the time-sensitive treatment may still be necessary if the patient is in extremis or unstable.

While the decision for diversion is ultimately up to the flight's captain, the responding clinician is often the best advocate for the patient at hand given their ability to physically assess the patient and their clinical expertise.

7.3 Management

Management of any in-flight medical emergency should begin with assessing the patient's vital signs and clinical stability. Airway protection in patients with decreased level of consciousness is typically considered for patients with a Glasgow

Coma Scale score equal to or less than 8 due to their decreased airway protective reflexes and increased risk of aspiration. However, the medical kit available on most commercial aircraft does not include endotracheal tubes or laryngoscopes; thus, one must consider alternative methods to reduce the risk of aspiration in these patients. One may consider leaving the patient upright in their seat or elevating their heads if their care is delivered on the floor. For patients who are hypoxic or at risk for cerebral hypoxia, supplemental oxygen may be provided, though it is limited to delivering 4–6 L/min of 100% oxygen [11]. One may consider requesting a descent to a lower altitude if there is evidence of respiratory distress or severe hypoxia not responsive to available oxygen delivery. If there are signs and symptoms of a herniation syndrome, hyperventilation of the patient can be performed using a bag valve mask.

Many neurological conditions require strict blood pressure management; however, given the lack of diagnostic certainty of in-flight neurological symptoms, simply avoiding hypotension and extreme hypertension would likely prevent secondary neurological injury and iatrogenic overtreatment. For the symptomatic hypotensive patients, intravenous access and fluids can be provided while epinephrine is available if there is concern for refractory shock. If a patient with stroke-like symptoms or altered mental status has extremely elevated blood pressure with systolic blood pressure greater than 220, few, if any, medications with antihypertensive effects are available in the onboard emergency medical kit. However, one should be cautious of potential labile responses to any blood pressure-augmenting medications given in a patient with in-flight neurological symptoms.

Blood glucose should be tested in patients with neurological symptoms given the propensity of hypo- and hyperglycemia to mimic neurological symptoms. While the medical kit available on aircraft does not typically contain a glucometer, passengers on the aircraft may have such equipment and may lend their device and supplies for flight staff use [12]. However, one must consider the potential for transmission of blood-borne pathogens.

7.3.1 Stroke

Stroke is a time-sensitive neurological emergency given the limited window for potential reperfusion therapies. Intravenous tissue plasminogen activator may be considered for patients with stroke-like symptoms should they meet eligibility criteria and are able to receive this therapy within 3–4.5 hours of symptom onset. Patients with symptoms of large vessel occlusion may be eligible for mechanical thrombectomy within 6 hours of symptom onset. Thus, in-flight stroke symptom is the most critical neurological emergency due to the limited time available in getting a patient to an appropriate facility for potential treatment.

Evaluation of a patient with in-flight stroke-like symptoms requires a detailed neurological exam to determine whether the symptoms are consistent with a vascular distribution. If symptoms are suggestive of a stroke, then discussion regarding the possibility of diversion should be initiated early with flight staff, pilots, and ground medical consultation so that they may begin evaluating whether diversion is logistically feasible.

Care of the patient with stroke-like symptoms should include close monitoring of vital signs and any change in their neurological exam. Supplemental oxygen should be provided to maintain oxygen saturation greater than 95% to reduce the risk of cerebral hypoxia. Hypoglycemia should be treated with oral or intravenous dextrose. While antiplatelet therapy with aspirin is indicated in acute ischemic stroke that is not a candidate for fibrinolysis or thrombectomy, given the limited diagnostic evaluation that can be performed to rule out intracranial hemorrhage, aspirin should not be administered for in-flight stroke-like symptoms.

7.3.2 Seizure

Seizures are usually self-limited; thus care of the seizing patient in-flight is usually supportive. Keeping the patient upright in their seat may reduce the risk of aspiration during a seizure; however, care should be provided to prevent the patient from head or limb injuries. Blood glucose should be tested in patients who seize during flight since hypoglycemia is an easily treatable cause of seizures.

For a single seizure that spontaneously resolves, care should include close monitoring of vital signs and return of the patient's mental status to baseline. Once the patient returns to baseline and if history is obtained that the patient has a known seizure disorder, one may recommend for the patient to take an additional dose of their prescribed seizure medication. If the patient does not return to baseline mental status and has recurrent or persistent seizures, then an anticonvulsant or sedative such as a benzodiazepine should be administered if available in the medical kit. Benzodiazepine may be administered intravenously or intramuscularly, depending on the availability of intravenous access. Diversion should be considered for patients with persistent or recurrent seizures, or prolonged alteration of mental status concerning for nonconvulsive seizures.

7.3.3 Altered Mental Status

Management of a patient with altered mental status in flight will be based on history and physical and is also largely supportive. Once again, blood glucose testing will be invaluable. Hypoxia, hypoventilation, and hypotension can all be treated with the available medical equipment on the aircraft. If the history supports intoxication or overdose, close monitoring of vital signs and the patient's neurological status will be key. Patients with altered mental status and focal neurological deficits should be considered for diversion for urgent definitive medical evaluation of potential intracranial hemorrhage.

The constellation of decline in mental status, asymmetric pupils, and posturing is consistent with a herniation event and should be treated emergently with hyperventilation with bag valve mask and establishment of intravenous access. While hyperventilation is typically used as a bridge to definitive treatment, treatment options are limited with the available medications in an aircraft's medical kit. If the patient has a known history of brain tumor, one may administer steroids for presumed vasogenic cerebral edema, though it is not recommended for nonneoplastic-related herniation events. If sodium bicarbonate is available in the medical kit, one may use it as a substitute for hypertonic saline given their similar osmolarity. An in-flight herniation event is a neurological emergency that needs to be diverted to a definitive medical facility. However, given the limited treatment options available on an aircraft, there is high likelihood of further deterioration of the patient into cardiac arrest.

7.3.4 Dizziness

The management of in-flight dizziness is generally supportive. Hypoglycemia and hypotension can be treated. Patients should be placed on cardiac monitoring if available to evaluate for possible arrhythmia. Nausea and vomiting associated with dizziness can be treated with the antiemetic available in the medical kit. Obtaining a detailed history of symptom onset and progression as well as utilizing the Head-Impulse-Nystagmus-Test-of-Skew (HINTS) exam will help differentiate between central causes such as vertebrobasilar insufficiency from peripheral causes such as labyrinthitis. If there is concern for vertebrobasilar insufficiency or posterior circulation stroke, diversion should be discussed with the flight staff, pilots, and ground medical consultation.

7.3.5 Headache

Analgesics are available in medical kits on aircraft and can be used for the treatment of headaches. However, aspirin and nonsteroidal anti-inflammatory drugs should be avoided if there is concern of an acute intracranial process such as subarachnoid hemorrhage or intracranial hemorrhage. Oxygen may be administered for tension-type headaches. Caffeinated beverages and intravenous fluids may be used to treat migraine-type headaches. Flight staff may also offer eye masks and earplugs if the patient is experiencing photophobia or phonophobia. Diversion should be considered if a patient with a headache has concomitant neurological deficits.

7.3.6 Head Injury

Most head injuries sustained in-flight are minor and may not require medical treatment. Analgesia and supportive care such as an ice pack may be provided. If the patient sustained a laceration from the traumatic injury, local wound care can be performed using drinking water or intravenous fluid to irrigate the wound. While basic dressing supplies such as gauze and tape are available in the medical kit on the aircraft, there is no equipment for laceration repair. If hemostasis cannot be achieved with direct pressure, one may consider using diluted epinephrine on the gauze to help local vasoconstriction within the wound. Achieving hemostasis of scalp lacerations is important as significant blood loss may occur given the highly vascular tissue.

7.4   Documentation

Documentation of in-flight neurological emergencies should include time of onset, duration of symptoms, as well as a detailed neurological assessment including level of consciousness, general language, and focality of any neurological deficits. Documentation forms may vary by airlines and may not include specific fields pertaining to neurological emergencies [13]. However, the more detail one is able to provide on the time course of the symptoms, the better prepared the receiving medical facility will be able to care for the patient.

Disclosure   The authors have nothing to disclose.

References

1. Urwin A, Ferguson J, McDonald R, Fraser S. A five-year review of ground-to-air emergency medical advice. J Telemed Telecare. 2008;14:157–9.
2. Sirven J, Claypool D, Sahs K, et al. Is there a neurologist on this flight? Neurology. 2002;58:1739–44.
3. Peterson DC, Martin-Gill C, Guyette FX, et al. Outcomes of medical emergencies on commercial airline flights. N Engl J Med. 2013;368:2075–83.
4. Pfausler B, Vollert H, Bosch S, Schmutzhard E. Cerebral venous thrombosis—a new diagnosis in travel medicine? J Travel Med. 1996;3:165–7.
5. Hughes R, Hopkins R, Hill S, et al. Frequency of venous thromboembolism in low to moderate risk long distance air travellers: the New Zealand Air Traveller's Thrombosis (NZATT) study. Lancet. 2003;362:2039–44.
6. Lapostolle F, Borron S, Surget V, Sordelet D, Lapandry C, Adnet F. Stroke associated with pulmonary embolism after air travel. Neurology. 2003;60:1983–5.
7. Leira EC, Cruz-Flores S, Wyrwich KW, et al. Improving pilot response to in-flight strokes: a randomized controlled trial. Cerebrovasc Dis. 2005;19:317–22.
8. Cummins RO, Schubach JA. Frequency and types of medical emergencies among commercial air travelers. JAMA. 1989;261:1296–9.
9. Hung KK, Chan EY, Cocks RA, Ong RM, Rainer TH, Graham CA. Predictors of flight diversions and deaths for in-flight medical emergencies in commercial aviation. Arch Intern Med. 2010;170:1401–2.
10. Muhm JM, Rock PB, McMullin DL, et al. Effect of aircraft-cabin altitude on passenger discomfort. N Engl J Med. 2007;357:18–27.
11. Rosenberg CA, Pak F. Emergencies in the air: problems, management, and prevention. J Emerg Med. 1996;15:159–64.
12. Nable JV, Tupe CL, Gehle BD, Brady WJ. In-flight medical emergencies during commercial travel. N Engl J Med. 2015;373:939–45.
13. Sand M, Morrosch S, Sand D, Altmeyer P, Bechara FG. Medical emergencies on board commercial airlines: is documentation as expected? Crit Care. 2012;16:R42.

Psychiatric Emergencies

8

Ryan Spangler

8.1 Introduction

The prospect of managing any patient in a resource-limited, closed environment can prove taxing, particularly when the environment is 35,000 ft in the air, and there are 100+ other persons onboard the aircraft. Anyone that has cared for patients experiencing an acute psychiatric issue has experienced the attendant difficulties in managing such patients, particularly if they are agitated or delirious. While such patients do not always have an immediate life-threatening concern, they can require a great deal of resources, even in a hospital setting, and can also be very disruptive to others in their vicinity. When these patients potentially have a concurrent life-threatening condition, as can happen perhaps more frequently than realized, their care becomes even more difficult. When psychiatric illness presents itself onboard an aircraft either alone or confounding another dangerous illness, the overhead page "Is there a doctor on board?" presents a unique challenge. The provider must take into account the safety of the patient at hand, as well as the safety of the other passengers onboard.

While little has been published overall on the subject, a few studies examine the incidence, causes, and treatment of in-flight psychiatric emergencies. One study found that about 3.5% of reported in-flight medical events are related to psychiatric emergencies, and 90% of these related to acute anxiety [1, 2]. Rarely do these circumstances require flight diversion, but many (69%) may require prompt evaluation upon landing at the flight's destination [2]. Furthermore, falling under the heading of psychiatric emergencies, it is also important to discuss behavioral emergencies including those such as the "air rage" phenomenon and otherwise intoxicated and/or angry passengers. In addition, there are several recognized psychiatric illnesses related to travel that, while maybe not directly related to the flight itself, can potentially present and be recognized in-flight.

R. Spangler, M.D.
Department of Emergency Medicine,
University of Maryland School of Medicine, Baltimore, MD, USA

© Springer International Publishing AG, part of Springer Nature 2018
J. V. Nable, W. Brady (eds.), *In-Flight Medical Emergencies*,
https://doi.org/10.1007/978-3-319-74234-2_8

8.2   Initial Approach

As with any condition, whether seen in the emergency department of a tertiary care hospital, or the passenger cabin of a mid-flight Boeing 747 passenger airliner, the initial evaluation of the patient should be focused on evaluating the safety of the environment, and then for an acute life-threatening emergency. Care needs to be taken not to overlook the possibility of an organic problem causing the patient's altered mental state, anxiety, or agitation. Patients presenting with anxiety could potentially be anxious due to true hypoxia, cardiac arrhythmia, or ischemia. Agitation, altered mental status, and confusion can all be caused by low blood sugar, and should not be missed. While the emergency medical kit (EMK) may not contain a blood glucose monitor or test strips, it is likely that another passenger may have one available to borrow (though the responding healthcare provider must be aware that cleanliness of borrowed devices cannot be ensured). If not, it is unlikely that empiric administration of oral or IV glucose (available in the EMK) is likely to worsen the patient's condition and may, in fact, improve it if hypoglycemia is the cause [3]. The use of orange juice, candy, or other food or beverage can also be used, provided that the patient can safely swallow. Evaluation of any patient should include a complete set of vital signs, if possible, as hypoxia may be apparent if a pulse oximeter is available. Although tachycardia is likely to be present in the anxious or agitated patient, extreme tachycardias may indicate the presence of atrial fibrillation or flutter with rapid ventricular response or supraventricular tachycardias.

8.3   Specific Illness

Many airlines have specific rules regarding travel of psychotic patients and generally require stabilization of the patient's mental state before allowing the person to fly. Airlines may even have the right to decline transport of passengers that they feel are unsafe to travel, which may limit the overall risk of psychotic behavior in-flight. This likely leads to an overwhelming number of psychiatric-related complaints onboard aircraft such as acute anxiety or panic attacks. Fortunately, these are rarely life-threatening. However, the specific patient's reaction may cause disruption of the flight for other passengers and, in severe cases, may actually put themselves or others at risk. For instance, an acutely agitated passenger may attempt to open doors or windows trying to escape. Angry and agitated passengers have also become a growing burden on the air travel industry.

8.3.1   Anxiety/Panic Disorder

Although firm definitions may not change treatment in this particular scenario, it is still relevant to discuss and use appropriate clinical terminology and disease definition. According to the Diagnostic and Statistical Manual of Mental Disorders (DSM)

Table 8.1 Anxiety disorders [4]

Separation anxiety disorder	Agoraphobia
Selective mutism	Generalized anxiety disorder
Specific phobia	Substance/medication-induced anxiety disorder
Social anxiety disorder (social phobia)	Anxiety disorder due to another medical condition
Panic disorder	Other specified anxiety disorder
Panic attack specifier	Unspecified anxiety disorder

Table 8.2 Symptoms of panic disorder [4]

Palpitations, pounding heart, accelerated heart rate	Sweating
Trembling or shaking	Sensations of shortness of breath or smothering
Feelings of choking	Chest pain or discomfort
Nausea or abdominal distress	Feeling dizzy, unsteady, lightheaded, or faint
Chills or heat sensations	Paresthesias
Derealization (feelings of unreality) or depersonalization (being detached from oneself)	Fear of losing control or "going crazy"
Fear of dying	–

V, multiple disorders are classified under Anxiety Disorders, including panic disorder (Table 8.1) [4]. This includes generalized anxiety disorder, social anxiety disorder, and specific phobias, all of which may contribute to an acute episode onboard an airplane. Many of the disorders in the anxiety spectrum are long-standing, and are centered around worry that tend to build over time and in certain situations. In this scenario, a person may show signs of nervousness from the beginning of the flight, that builds throughout the flight, with or without a specific trigger for worsening [4].

Panic disorder is a specific subcategory in the "Anxiety Disorders" and occurs in 2–3% of the population in adolescents and adults, particularly among the Caucasian and European population [5, 6]. Generally, rates tend to increase in adolescents and decline in older patients [6, 7]. Women tend to be affected more than men (2:1) and prepubescent children have a very low rate of true panic disorder [5].

A panic attack, by definition, generally occurs very abruptly and is often unexpected. The patient may fear having a panic attack and avoid certain situations that they know may trigger an attack. DSM V criteria for panic attack defines the illness as an abrupt surge of intense fear or intense discomfort that reaches a peak within minutes and during which time 4 (or more) specific symptoms occur (Table 8.2) [4]. In order to diagnose panic disorder, an attack must be followed by 1 month or more of worry about the event, worrying it may recur and the consequences, and/or "maladapative changes" to avoid another event [4]. The presentation of a panic attack can be potentially a difficult situation to handle in a limited in-flight environment, as many of the symptoms listed have significant overlap with life-threatening illness. Respiratory, cardiac, and metabolic abnormalities can all present with tachycardia, shortness of breath, and feeling faint, for example. It is important for the physician in these cases to carefully take the patient's history, medical conditions, medications, and presentation into account to consider the need for further evaluation to rule out other life-threatening conditions.

8.3.2   Air Rage

"Air rage" is hardly a new phenomenon, but one that has become increasingly prevalent and has received significant media coverage. Although frequently it does not involve a "medical" complaint, cabin crew may require or request assistance and intervention. Air rage refers to unruly, agitated, and potentially aggressive behavior, both physically and verbally, that seems to arise from circumstances surrounding air travel. According to the Washington Post, the number of reported events from 2015 increased by over 1,500 from 2014, resulting in a reported episode in approximately 1 per 1,200 flights [8]. There have been smaller observational studies addressing this issue that have attempted to identify contributing factors to increased agitation and aggressive behavior.

Recent incidents from the news:

- NBC reported a flight that was forced to return to the airport in New York in order to have an unruly passenger removed [9].
- Metro UK reported that a pilot tackled a drunk passenger that had allegedly assaulted a flight attendant [10].
- DailyMail.com reported a video of agitated patient arguing with flight attendant over two plastic cups [11].
- 7 ABC News Denver reported approximately 200 calls for disturbances onboard aircraft called to Denver International Airport from 2011 to 2012 [12].
- NBCNews.com details an incident involving an Icelandair passenger restrained with duct tape after the drunken male became disruptive en route to JFK International airport in New York in 2013 [13].

Many contributing, or inciting, events seem to be related to typical, obvious stress- and frustration-inducing scenarios. Flight delays, cancellations, overbooking, and alcohol consumption generally seem to increase passenger agitation [14, 15]. Diminishing seat size (both width and pitch) has also been suggested to be a contributing factor to conflict between passengers. This has not been shown definitively to lead to increased air rage, but the steady decline of seat sizes and space tends to be associated with the steady increase in the incidence of air rage, as well as passenger perception of their own anxiety and agitation [14].

One study also looked at air rage as a product of social inequality. The study found that separate "statuses" such as first class and economy lead to an increase in air rage, not only in the economy class, but also in the first-class cabin. Factors such as front-of-plane boarding (vs. middle), requiring passengers to walk through first class to reach economy, can increase the number of air rage incidents [15]. Agitated types of behavior amounted largely to both belligerent behavior and intoxication-related complaints, and had a large male preponderance. Incidents mostly occurred in the economy class (84%). Comparing first-class incidents with those in economy class, behavior resulting from a passenger's strong anger occurred in a larger percent in the first-class incidents, while incidents related to emotional outburst tended to occur in a large percent in the economy class. The authors hypothesized that the visual representation of their social inequalities, both advantaged and disadvantaged passengers, may lead to increased anger and lack of emotional control. Less incidents tended to occur on flights that did not have first-class seating [15].

8.3.3 Psychosis

Interestingly, there are several types of psychoses that may be specifically related to travel. Not all are associated with the in-flight portion of the travel; however, the psychotic behavior may present itself en route to a destination, or at the destination, and may or may not persist while leaving the destination, and therefore may be encountered in-flight. Generic terms such as "travel-induced psychosis" have been applied, indicating a new psychiatric episode or psychosis in patients due to traveling abroad. This phenomenon is often seen in young adults, but even the elderly may be susceptible [16]. Treatment in-flight for any of these conditions may not change from management of any other psychotic condition; however, familiarity with the syndromes may make a responding provider more comfortable assessing the situation should one be asked to evaluate a passenger potentially experiencing an acute psychotic event.

Even more specific psychoses, such as "Jerusalem syndrome," have also been identified. Jerusalem syndrome has been suggested as a psychosis specifically related to traveling to the city of Jerusalem. Interestingly, this can occur in both travelers with previous mental health illness and those that are previously completely healthy, and sometimes completely healthy after return from Jerusalem. Three "types" have been delineated for this particular syndrome. In some cases, the impetus to travel to Jerusalem may be part of a preexisting delusional psychotic belief (type 1). However, other cases result in psychosis after spending time in the city. These patients can be lone travelers, or in groups. The second type may not display florid psychosis or easily definable delusions, but may have obsession with a fixed idea and strange thoughts. The final group is perhaps the most interesting. This includes patients previously completely medically and psychiatrically healthy prior to travel, who develop clearly progressing psychosis while in Jerusalem. The condition, in this final group, usually resolves with conservative or no treatment, within days after removal or distancing the patient from the city itself [17].

8.4   Treatment Options

8.4.1   Anxiety/Panic

In many cases, the only treatment needed may be reassurance and time. In other situations, calming exercises such as deep breathing, lying down, or loosening any tight clothing may be beneficial. It has been suggested that the acute attacks associated with panic disorder may have a respiratory trigger and that focused breathing training may help patients deal with these attacks [18]. Feelings of breathlessness, which may potentially be caused by lower oxygen concentrations at high altitude of flight, could potentially trigger this mechanism, although this specific cause has not been studied. Some limited studies have investigated the theory that increased sensitivity to concentrations of carbon dioxide in the bloodstream may be a cause of panic attacks in some patients triggering hyperventilation. Theories from the 1980s suggest that the hyperventilatory response in a panic attack causes a positive feedback loop, in which the patient feels more and more uncomfortable due to the symptoms associated with respiratory alkalosis, which further exacerbates the attack [19]. The patients also have been postulated to respond to physiologic hyperventilation as a life-threatening event, rather than a normal physiologic correction [20].

While long-term cognitive behavioral therapy is the basis of treatment for those with panic disorder, the theories discussed above have led to the introduction of breathing training as a technique to handle acute panic. This typically focuses on teaching the patient to recognize that hyperventilation at times is a normal response, and not life threatening. Unfortunately, due to varying study designs, small sample sizes, and inconsistent results, the overall validity of the hyperventilation theory, increased carbon dioxide blood concentration sensitivity, and overall utility of breathing training remain unconfirmed. In the acute setting, however, without other resources available, attempts to help the patient calm their breathing, potentially to restore normal carbon dioxide levels, may be beneficial [21]. This can be achieved with simple coaching to help the patient slow breathing and decrease minute ventilation, or with the assistance of bag rebreathing if necessary. Care must be taken, however, if the patient's anxiety is caused by hypoxia, as bag breathing can further reduce oxygen blood concentration levels, and has even reportedly led to death if inappropriately applied [22].

In cases in which these techniques are ineffective, the emergency medical kit on board is also unlikely to be particularly helpful. The contents required by the FAA contain no ideal option for a rapidly sedating medication, with the exception of an "antihistamine medication" (most likely diphenhydramine), in both oral and injectable routes [23]. The requirement to carry these medications is surely in order to treat the possibility of an anaphylactic reaction, but may be repurposed for sedation if the situation requires. It would certainly be prudent to weigh the risks and benefits of utilizing this antihistamine medication (particularly the IV/IM route) which also has anticholinergic properties. In many cases, a passenger may already have a known diagnosis of anxiety or panic attacks and may be carrying his or her personal medications specifically for this purpose.

8.4.2   Agitated Patients

Handling of these agitated patients does not, in theory, require the specific assistance of a medical provider. However, it may be necessary to intervene, and medical assistance may be requested to determine if there is a medical/psychiatric component to the agitated behavior, particularly if it is due to agitated psychosis. If less restrictive methods to calm and reassure the patient fail, it may be necessary to sedate and/or restrain the patient. As previously discussed, there are limited options for pharmacological sedation.

Initial attempts to address agitated behavior should begin with verbal de-escalation of the situation. Attempting to confront the patient aggressively, in a dominant-submissive manner, as if one were disciplining a child, may potentially escalate the passenger's agitation and aggression. A consensus statement from an emergency psychiatry de-escalation workgroup describes a potentially successful technique that allows the patient to participate in calming and gain internal control of their emotions. The three stages of de-escalation described are to first verbally engage the patient, then establish a collaborative relationship, and finally de-escalate the patient from the agitated state. The group identifies ten "domains" of de-escalation that can help improve the interaction and the success of the interaction (Table 8.3) [24].

Many airlines may have a supply of emergency restraints available to help deal with dangerous passengers if required. If not, it may be necessary to request assistance of other passengers and crew members to creatively and safely devise a method to restrain a patient. While rarely necessary, one may worry about the legal ramifications, both criminal and civil, when attempting to restrain an unwilling passenger on

Table 8.3 De-escalation techniques [24]

Domains of de-escalation	Key recommendation
Respect personal space	Maintain two arms-lengths of distance. This provides patient and provider safety distance for exit if needed
Do not be provocative	Use calm language and tone, and safe body language
Establish verbal contact	Only one person should verbally interact with the patient. Introduce yourself and provide reassurance that you want to help them
Be concise	Short, simple phrasing and word choice
Identify wants and feelings	Use "free information" to identify. Patients mood, affect, and body language can help identify their goals
Listen closely to what the patient is saying	Actively listen and use clarifying statements
Agree or agree to disagree	Use of "fogging" to identify aspect of patient's position with which you can both agree
Lay down the law and set clear limits	Establish clear working conditions matter of factly, not a threat
Offer choices and optimism	Offer realistic choices and alternatives to aggression or fight or flight; this helps the patient not feel trapped
Debrief the patient and staff	Reestablish therapeutic relationship with the patient after any involuntary action is taken

board an airplane. The Tokyo Convention in 1963 outlined a pilot and airline crew's right to restrain and utilize passenger assistance in the event that it is felt the passenger may be a danger to the flight or other passengers [25]. This stance was reaffirmed with the Montreal Protocol of 2014 as well [26]. International Air Transport Association (IATA) protocols dictate that able-bodied passengers may be requested to assist with restraining an unruly passenger if they become physically threatening or are felt to be a danger to themselves or others on the flight. It is not mandatory to assist with restraints, and the cabin crew should dictate the procedure, and not relinquish control to passengers, regardless of profession [27]. If restraints are not available aboard the flight, more creative measures may have to be taken to control an unruly passenger. Reports of other passengers supplying duct tape, belts, ties, etc. to be used to restrain an aggressive and/or intoxicated individual have occurred. Reportedly only a minority, about 11–17%, of cases of unruly passengers opened by the FAA actually result in prosecution of the offending passenger [28].

8.4.3   Suicide

In a clinical setting, evaluating a patient's risk of suicide is often one of the primary goals when initially assessing a psychiatric patient. If one were to encounter a potentially suicidal passenger in flight, it will be necessary to maintain the safety of the patient and other passengers by any of the mechanisms previously described. If the person had attempted to harm themselves, stabilizing treatment for any injuries may be required.

Few studies have investigated aircraft-assisted suicides committed by pilots. This is, however, a very uncommon event (16 of 3,648 fatal aviation accidents) [29]. When flying onboard commercial aircraft as a passenger, there is, however, frequently very little contact or access to the pilot in order to assess the situation, even if there were early warning signs. In 50% of the cases referenced above, pilots tested positive for illicit substances [29]. In the event that a copilot or other crew member had concerns for the pilot's mental state, and ask for physician assistance, it may be reasonable to have another capable crew member take over and have the pilot further evaluated upon landing.

Conclusion

While psychiatric complaints continue to make up only a small portion of medical complaints aboard aircraft, the vast number of daily flights and increasing number of passengers aboard these flights make it likely that at some point a physician may be requested to assess one of these passenger-patients. Perhaps even more likely, an ever-increasing trend of "air rage" and unruly passengers seems to exist. Dealing with any of these situations can be difficult. While pharmacologic support may be limited, focused breathing, verbal de-escalation, and, if necessary, physical restraint may be required. After ruling out and/or treating potential underlying medical causes of any symptoms, hopefully the suggested techniques listed in this chapter may aid in the assessment and treatment of any illness or disruption.

References

1. Peterson DC, Martin-Gill C, Guyette FX, Tobias AZ, McCarthy CE, Harrington ST, et al. Outcomes of medical emergencies on commercial airline flights. N Engl J Med. 2013;368:2075–83. https://doi.org/10.1056/NEJMoa1212052.
2. Matsumoto K, Goebert D. In-flight psychiatric emergencies. Aviat Space Environ Med. 2001;72(10):919–23.
3. Federal Aviation Administration (FAA), Department of Transportation. Emergency medical equipment: final rule. Fed Regist. 2001;66:19028–46.
4. American Psychiatric Association. Diagnostic and statistical manual of mental disorders, 5th ed. 2013.
5. Goodwin RD, Faravelli C, Rosi S, Cosci F, Truglia E, de Graaf R, Wittchen HU. The epidemiology of panic disorder and agoraphobia in Europe. Eur Neuropsychopharmacol. 2005;15(4):435–43.
6. Kessler RC, Petukhova M, Sampson NA, Zaslavsky AM, Wittchen HU. Twelve-month and lifetime prevalence and lifetime morbid risk of anxiety and mood disorders in the United States. Int J Methods Psychiatr Res. 2012;21(3):169–84. https://doi.org/10.1002/mpr/1359.
7. Craske MG, Kircanski K, Epstein A, Wittchen HU, Pine DS, Lewis-Fernández R, Hinton D. Panic disorder: a review of DSM-IV panic disorder and proposals for DSM-V. Depress Anxiety. 2010;27(2):93–112.
8. International Air Transport Association (IATA). Collaboration Needed To Stem Unruly Passenger Incidents. 2016. http://www.iata.org/pressroom/pr/Pages/2016-09-28-01.aspx. Accessed 1 Dec 2016.
9. Holt S, Cheng P. Flight returns to JFK to Remove 'Disruptive" Passenger: Officials. In: NBC 4 New York. 14 Sept 2016. http://www.nbcnewyork.com/news/local/Flight-Returns-to-Kennedy-Airport-Disruptive-Passenger-Plane-American-Airlines-393333621.html. Accessed 13 Dec 2016.
10. Nsubuga J. Pilot forced to restrain 'drunk' passenger who just wouldn't sit down. In: Metro.co.uk. 2 Aug 2016. http://metro.co.uk/2016/08/02/pilot-forced-to-restrain-drunk-passenger-who-just-wouldnt-sit-down-6043463/. Accessed 13 Dec 2016.
11. Farberov S. 'This is all about two plastic cups': Spirit Airlines passenger's in-flight meltdown is caught on camera. In: Dailymail.com. 15 Aug 2016. http://www.dailymail.co.uk/news/article-3741934/This-two-plastic-cups-Spirit-Airlines-passenger-s-flight-meltdown-caught-camera.html. Accessed 13 Dec 2016.
12. Unruly Airline Passenger Incidents Growing. In: ABC 7 Denver. 22 Aug 2012. http://www.thedenverchannel.com/news/unruly-airline-passenger-incidents-growing. Accessed 13 Dec 2016.
13. Diaz L. How flight attendants deal with unruly passengers travel on NBCNews.com. In: YouTube.com. https://www.youtube.com/watch?v=cZKKZaPKbmM. Accessed 2 Dec 2016.
14. Vredenburgh AN, Zackowitz IB, Vredenburgh AG. Air Rage: what factors influence airline passenger anger? In: Proceedings of the Human Factors and Ergonomics Society 59th annual meeting; 2015. p. 400–4.
15. DeCelles KA, Norton MI. Physical and situational inequality on airplanes predicts air rage. Proc Natl Acad Sci U S A. 2016;113(20):5588–91. https://doi.org/10.1073/pnas.1521727113.
16. Felkai P, Kurimay T. The most vulnerable travelers: patients with mental disorders. World Psychiatry. 2011;10(3):237.
17. Bar-El Y, Durst R, Katz G, Zislin J, Strauss Z, Knobler HY. Jerusalem syndrome. Br J Psychiatry. 2000;176:86–90. https://doi.org/10.1192/bjp.176.1.86.
18. Meuret AE, Wilhelm FH, Roth WT. Respiratory biofeedback-assisted therapy in panic disorder. Behav Modif. 2001;25(4):584–605.
19. Clark D A cognitive approach to panic. Behav Res Ther 1986;24(4):461–70.
20. Ley R. The many faces of Pan: psychological and physiological differences amount three types of panic attacks. Behav Res Ther 199230(4):347–57.

21. Meuret AE, Wilhelm FH, Ritz T, Roth WT. Breathing Training for Treating Panic disorder: useful intervention or impediment? Behav Modif. 2003;27(5):731–54.
22. Callaham M. Hypoxic hazards of traditional paper bag rebreathing in hyperventilating patients. Ann Emerg Med. 1989;18(6):622–8.
23. Vancouver Coastal Health: Formulary: Therapuetic Tools. (2016). http://www.vhpharmsci.com/vhformulary/Tools/Tools-Index.htm. Accessed 12 Dec 2016.
24. Richmond JS, Berlin JS, Fishkind AB, Holloman Jr GH, Zeller SJ, Wilson MP, et al. Verbal de-escalation of the agitated patient: consensus statement of the American Association for Emergency Psychiatry Project BETA de-escalation workgroup. West J Emerg Med 2012;13(1):17–25. doi:https://doi.org/10.5811/westjem.2011.9.6864.
25. International Civil Aviation Organization (ICAO). Convention on Offences and Certain Other Acts Committed on Board Aircraft. International Conference on Air Law. Tokyo; 1963.
26. International Civil Aviation Organization (ICAO). Protocol to Amend the Convention on Offences and Certain Other Acts Commited on Board Aircraft. Montréal; 2014.
27. International Air Transport Association (IATA). Guidance on Unruly Passenger Prevention and Management. 2015 Jan. 2nd edition.
28. Stock S, Villareal M, Nious K. Chaos on commercial flights: unruly airline passengers rarely face criminal charges. In: NBC Bay Area 15 Dec 2015. http://www.nbcbayarea.com/investigations/Unruly-Passengers-Escape-Prosecution-362016541.html. Accessed 15 Dec 2016.
29. Lewis RJ, Johnson RD, Whinnery JE, Forster EM. Aircraft-assisted pilot suicides in the United States, 1993–2002. Arch Suicide Res 2007;11(2):149–61.

Pediatric Considerations

9

Kathleen Stephanos

9.1 Overview

Pediatric patients require special consideration. Aside from different physiology and age-specific medical conditions, medications must be dosed based on weight to avoid overdosing the patient. Several of the FAA-required onboard medications are rarely utilized in pediatrics and some are contraindicated. Additionally, medications available on flights are rarely in liquid formulation, making these much more difficult to dose in an austere environment.

Fortunately, pediatric in-flight emergencies occur at a significantly lower rate than those of adults. Pediatric emergencies comprise approximately 11% of all in-flight medical events [1, 2]. The most common ailments encountered include gastrointestinal, infectious, neurologic, allergic, and respiratory illnesses [1]. This chapter reviews the special considerations of the neonate, pediatric-specific responses to a variety of conditions, how to estimate weight, and utilization of accessible resources including altering the available supplies to accommodate a smaller patient.

When dealing with children, it is crucial to remember that a factor in pediatric emergencies is also management of the parent or guardian who is present. This individual is a responding provider's resource for most, if not all, of the medical history and description of the events leading up to the present need for medical attention. Helping to calm a parent may play more of a role in patient care than the care of the patient alone.

K. Stephanos, M.D.
Department of Emergency Medicine, Strong Memorial Hospital, Rochester, NY, USA
e-mail: Kathleen_Stephanos@urmc.rochester.edu

© Springer International Publishing AG, part of Springer Nature 2018
J. V. Nable, W. Brady (eds.), *In-Flight Medical Emergencies*,
https://doi.org/10.1007/978-3-319-74234-2_9

9.2   The Neonate

A ground-based consultation service that provides medical advice to approximately 10% of global air traffic has reported in-flight labor and delivery to occur approximately 5 times per year [3]. While this is a rare occurrence, the infants born in this setting are at higher risk than a typical birth. For delivery-related treatment, please see Chap. 10 on obstetrics. Often, these deliveries are precipitous and may result in a premature infant. Many airlines will not allow women who are >36 wks gestation to fly (earlier on some longer flights), though they may or may not require documentation to board the aircraft [2]. Presuming that patients are aware of their pregnancy, know their dates accurately, and are truthful in reporting, most in-flight deliveries will be preterm infants resulting in a different list of complications to be considered in the minutes following delivery. Neonates (<3 mos of age) are managed very differently from other children [4].

9.2.1   APGAR Scoring

Initial assessment of any neonate is based predominantly on appearance. A well-appearing infant is likely healthy. The APGAR scoring system is the generally accepted method to assess a neonate's need for intervention [5].

APGAR scoring is completed at 1, 5, and 10 min postdelivery (10 min is only necessary if APGAR is <9 at 5 min or there is a clinical change). Table 9.1 demonstrates the five assessed features in the APGAR score, along with associated points [5]. This is used as a general assessment of neonatal transition. Most commonly, well infants will have persistent acrocyanosis (extremities that are blue or cyanotic), and this can be normal in an otherwise-well infant until 12 mos of age. This means that healthy infants rarely receive a score higher than 9.

It is important to note that APGAR scoring is used for a general assessment of infant health, has several more subjective measures, and has not been proven to directly correlate with overall outcomes unless extremely low (<3) [6].

Table 9.1 APGAR scoring system, used for general newborn assessment [5]

	Points		
	0	1	2
Activity (tone)	None	Flexed extremities	Moving extremities
Pulse (beats/min)	None	<100	>100
Grimace	None	Grimace	Sneeze, cough, moves away
Appearance (color)	Blue	Pink centrally, blue extremities	Pink
Respirations	None	Irregular, slow	Regular

9.2.2 Neonatal Resuscitation of the Full-Term Infant

A full-term infant is defined as an infant who has complete 37 wks (approximately 8.5 mos) of gestation. In the full-term infant, the primary goals following delivery are stimulating the infant and providing warmth. In an austere environment, warmth can be provided most effectively by drying the infant quickly and as thoroughly as possible, then allowing the bare infant to be placed directly on his or her mother's skin, allowing for direct transfer of heat. Clothing should be covering the area not in contact with skin. This is particularly important during flights where the ambient temperature is typically 19–23 °C (66.2–73.4 °F) with low humidity of 6–14%, resulting in rapid cooling and evaporative losses for an infant [2].

Of the vital signs in a neonate, the heart rate will most directly influence management. If an infant appears cyanotic, is breathing, and has a normal heart rate above 100 beats/min, blow-by oxygen (or air) can be given to improve perfusion. Once pink, a trial without oxygen supplementation should be performed. Restarting oxygen is appropriate if the infant becomes dusky or cyanotic again. If initial blow-by therapy does not improve color, positive-pressure ventilation is indicated. The mask does not require oxygen to be effective—air alone can be used. Oxygen in excess has been shown to be detrimental to neonates, and should not be over-utilized.

Apnea or heart rate below 100 beats/min at 30 s of life should prompt immediate positive-pressure ventilation using a bag valve mask. Heart rate less than 60 beats/min at 1 min of life indicates the need to initiate cardiopulmonary resuscitation (CPR). CPR in a neonate is ideally provided by 2 providers, with one at the foot of the patient with 2 thumbs placed on the sternum and the remaining fingers wrapped around the back. Compressions should be at a ratio of 3 compressions for each breath. Another method is for the provider to use an index and middle finger on the sternum for compressions. Due to the high ratio of 3 compressions for every 1 breath, there is limited utility in attempting this alone.

If a pulse oximeter is available, it is important to note that a neonate's oxygen will not reach >90% until over 10 min of age. Initial oxygen levels at 1 min are typically 60% due to shifts in vascular flow and gradually increase to 85% over the first 10 min of life. This makes pulse oximeter readings a poor tool for assessment of resuscitation status of a neonate. Oxygen saturation measurements should always be obtained on the right hand, resulting in a preductal saturation. This is an important feature, as providing unnecessary oxygen can result in retinal issues, and positive pressure can result in a pneumothorax if used too vigorously.

A vigorous infant, who appears well after delivery, is warm, breathing without grunting, pink, and able to nurse, may not warrant an expedited landing unless there are concerns for the mother's health [4].

9.2.3 Neonatal Resuscitation of the Preterm Infant

Preterm infant birth often requires additional resuscitative efforts. Infants between 29 and 37 wks of gestation may be approached in a similar manner to a full-term infant, with particular care taken to keep these infants warm.

Infants less than 29 wks of gestation have much higher evaporative cooling losses, and rather than immediate drying should be wrapped in plastic with any external warmth available applied to the infant. Food-grade plastic wrap is appropriate with only the face left exposed. Again, the mother's skin may be the best source of warmth; a blanket covering a heating pad may be of assistance. There is some evidence that this may be useful in neonates up to 34 wks gestation and should be considered, particularly if the ambient temperature is low, as is common on commercial flights [7]. Respiratory compromise is extremely likely in this age range due to underdeveloped lung tissue. Gentle positive-pressure oxygenation may be needed, with the smallest available mask. It may be necessary to turn an infant-size mask upside down (narrower nose portion placed on the chin) to obtain an appropriate seal. Delivery of a premature infant should prompt consideration for early landing, if possible.

Again, heart rate is used to determine the need for respiratory or cardiac interventions. A heart rate of less than 100 beats/min at 30 s of life is an indication for positive-pressure ventilation. A heart rate of less than 60 beats/min after 1 min is an indication to begin chest compressions. CPR is provided in a ratio of 3 compressions to 1 breath with 2 providers.

Infants less than 23 wks of gestation have limited survival in ideal settings and exhaustive resuscitation should not be performed. In these cases, care should be focused on the mother [4].

9.3   The General Pediatric Patient

9.3.1   Respiratory Issues

The most common cause of significant pediatric illness and mortality that may occur in flight is respiratory distress. Respiratory failure is the most common cause of cardiac arrest in children [8]. The anatomy of a pediatric airway is distinctly different from that of an adult. The trachea is shorter and narrower, characterized by an anterior pharynx and narrow cricothyroid membrane. Tonsils are also larger, resulting in potential obstruction. Children typically have a much larger occiput than adults and may require more manipulation to allow an airway to be patent [9]. Responding providers should consider utilizing neck rolls (fabric rolled and placed under the shoulders to elevate the neck), and ensure that the ear is at the level of the sternal notch without hyperextending or flexing the neck to keep an airway open for pediatric patients experiencing respiratory arrest. Respiratory rates are expected to be higher in children than adults (see Table 9.2) [8].

Asthma. Asthma is one of the most common chronic illnesses of pediatrics with over 6 million US children living with asthma. The medical management of asthma is, fortunately, the same for adults and children. A patient will often present with subcostal, supraclavicular, or intra-costal retractions, with nasal flaring and expiratory wheezing. Younger children often have more dramatic retractions than older children or adults. In severe cases, only decreased breath sounds may be heard, with

Table 9.2 Weight estimations and vital signs based on age [8]

Age	Estimated weight (lbs)	Estimated weight (kg)	Heart rate (beats/min)	Low systolic blood pressure (mmHg)	Respiratory rate (breaths/min)
Neonate	7.5	3.5	85–160	60	40–60
1–2 months	11	5	85–160	70	30–60
3–4 months	17	8	75–190	70	30–60
5–6 months	22	10	75–190	70	30–60
7–11 months	24	11	75–190	70	30–60
1 year	26	12	75–190	72	24–40
2 years	30	14	75–190	74	24–40
3 years	35	16	60–140	76	22–34
4 years	40	18	60–140	78	22–34
5 years	44	20	60–140	80	18–30
6 years	52	24	60–140	82	18–30
7 years	61	28	60–140	84	18–30
8 years	70	32	60–140	86	18–30
9 years	79	36	60–140	88	18–30
10 years	88	40	60–140	90	12–16
11 years	97	44	50–100	90	12–16
12 years	105	48	50–100	90	12–16
13 years	114	52	50–100	90	12–16
14 years	123	56	50–100	90	12–16
>14 years	132	60	50–100	90	12–16

These are estimates and clinical judgment should be used to avoid overdosing medications. Weight in pounds is included to help in cases where parents know the child's weight, but should never be used for calculating doses. For patient safety, if you know the child's weight and it is between two weight groups, use the lower number

or without faint wheezing. A bronchodilator, typically albuterol, is the first-line therapy. Dosing is identical for adults and children and can be administered via nebulizer or metered-dose inhaler (MDI). If only an MDI is readily available, a spacer will allow for more medication to reach the lung tissue [10, 11]. This can be helpful in all age groups for optimization of medication, but is especially important in children who are unable to coordinate inhalation with medication release. On a commercial aircraft, a foam or plastic cup can be used to aide in administration. A hole is made in the cup's bottom and the mouthpiece of the MDI placed within the hole. Puffs of the MDI are administered while the cup's rim is applied to the face and held in place for 10 s (repeat for each puff individually). In severe exacerbations of asthma, 10 puffs every hour is appropriate. If this alone does not improve symptoms, other medications on board may be useful. If steroids are available, they may be given. Otherwise, anaphylactic dosing of intramuscular epinephrine should be considered for patients in extremis [11, 12].

Anaphylaxis. Allergic reaction is common in all patient populations, but particularly in children, with the most common allergies being to peanuts, milk, and tree nuts. Five to six percent of all children have a food allergy. Insects, medications, or environmental exposures, such as latex, may also result in an allergic reaction. Patients may not always know that they have an allergy prior to anaphylaxis. The recognition of anaphylactic symptoms, along with prompt treatment with epinephrine, is essential. Anaphylaxis should be considered if 2 or more organ systems are involved with symptoms—gastrointestinal, dermatologic, respiratory, or cardiovascular. This can present in many different ways—wheezing, vomiting, diarrhea, syncope, lightheadedness, shortness of breath, hives, mouth or throat swelling, sneezing, irritability, eye itching or tearing, or a drop in blood pressure. Epinephrine can be given repeatedly every 10–15 min as needed to stabilize. Epinephrine should be 1:1,000 concentration, with children less than 30 kg receiving 0.15 mg, and those weighing greater than 30 kg receiving 0.3–0.5 mg IM epinephrine injected into the lateral thigh. This can be done through clothing if needed. Adjuncts to this include diphenhydramine (1 mg/kg IV or PO), IV fluids (20 mL/kg bolus), albuterol, and steroids when available [13].

Croup. Croup is a common cause of respiratory distress in young children (often <2 years of age). It presents with inspiratory stridor, a brassy or "barking seal-like" cough. The ideal treatment is steroids if available, ideally dexamethasone given its long half-life. Nebulized racemic epinephrine can also improve symptoms, if available. Nebulized epinephrine can also be used, and can be created by mixing 1:10,000 2.5–5 mL with 3 mL saline added into the nebulizer. Unfortunately, these medications are less likely to be available aboard a commercial flight, so placing the child in a position of comfort, often in a tripod position with head in a sniffing position, and providing oxygen, if available, may help. The cool air of the cabin may be in the patient's favor in this situation [14].

Foreign bodies. Due to the differences in pediatric airways as well as their not unusual interest in putting items in their mouths, children are at higher risk for aspiration and foreign-body airway obstruction. Common items that become lodged in the airway include nuts, vegetables, fruits, toys, and pins [15]. Appropriate response to this situation depends on age. A patient that can breathe or speak should be encouraged to cough, but no other maneuvers should be attempted. The Heimlich maneuver (abdominal thrusts), while lifesaving, is not without risks, including abdominal or thoracic trauma [16]. In children under 1 yr of age, 5 back blows should be given with the child's body across the thigh of the provider and the head lower to the ground than the body. The child should then be turned to a supine position, head down and supported, and 5 abdominal thrusts using 2 fingers applied just below the sternum should be provided. In older children and adults, the traditional "Heimlich maneuver" should be used with 5 back blows followed by 5 abdominal thrusts with 2 hands clasped and applied just below the sternum. It is important not to do blind finger sweeps to prevent pushing an item further into the airway. If a patient becomes unresponsive, the responding provider should look for an object in the airway and begin rescue breaths [17].

Pneumothorax. A pneumothorax can occur in flight due, in part, to pressure changes in the cabin. It should also be in the differential for a newborn infant who suddenly worsens, especially after receiving positive-pressure ventilation. Treatment is based on the severity of symptoms. In patients with pneumothorax who have significant respiratory distress, the placement of a large-bore needle into the anterior chest wall's second intercostal space in the midclavicular line on the side of the chest without breath sounds may result in air release. Patients should be placed on supplemental oxygen if available. Patients without significant distress can be placed on oxygen when available and have repeat examinations. The cabin pressure changes can worsen a pneumothorax, making this a high-risk condition for decompensating [18].

9.3.2   Cardiac Issues

Assessing cardiovascular status. The sphygmomanometer provided in the emergency medical kit is unlikely the correct size for a child. Due to the cuff being large, it will have limited utility in a small child; it will likely report falsely low blood pressures. A better marker of perfusion is capillary refill time of the extremities, which should be less than 2–3 s in a healthy patient. Heart rate is also important in pediatric cardiac assessment. Tachycardia will persist for longer in children than adults before hypotension occurs. If an accurate blood pressure can be obtained, the following calculation can be used to help identify normal blood pressures:

Systolic blood pressure = $[70 + (age \times 2)]$

Below this level should indicate hypotension.

Typically boluses of intravenous (IV) fluids are approximately 20 cm^3/kg, as long as the patient has no known cardiac illness or renal issues, causing increased risk for fluid overload. If long-term care is expected in-flight due to inability to land, maintenance fluids can be calculated based on weight [8]:

– First 10 kg give 4 mL/kg/h
– Second 10 kg give 2 mL/kg/h (in addition to above)
– Beyond 20 kg give 1 mL/kg/h (in addition to above)
– For example, a 32 kg child would receive:
  4 mL/h for the first 10 kg = 40 mL/h
  2 mL/h for the second 10 kg = 20 mL/h
  1 mL/h for the remaining kg = 2 mL/h
  Total = 62 mL/h

Cardiac arrest. If a child has poor perfusion, is unresponsive despite appropriate oxygenation, and has a heart rate less than 60 beats/min, CPR should be started. If the patient has no pulse, CPR should also be initiated at a rate of 15 compressions followed by 2 breaths, with a goal of 100 compressions per min. Epinephrine should be given IV 1:10,000 concentration 0.01 mg/kg every 3–5 min.

Automated external defibrillators (AEDs) should be available on most commercial flights. Ideally, both adult and pediatric pads will be stocked. If only adult pads are present, the responding provider may place the right chest wall pad onto the child's back in the midline of the upper back, and the left chest wall pad placed anterior to the child's heart [8].

Chest pain. Cardiac issues are extremely rare in children and often have been diagnosed prior to flight. Unlike in adults, chest pain is more likely to be related to respiratory causes than cardiac, therefore aspirin is not typically indicated. Aspirin is contraindicated in children due to the potential for the development of Reye's syndrome. Nitroglycerin has virtually no indication in children. Pediatric chest pain patients should have a cardiac and lung examination with palpation of the chest. It is important to assess for wheezing, decreased breath sounds, or stridor. Chest wall tenderness may respond to acetaminophen or ibuprofen [19].

Supraventricular tachycardia. Supraventricular tachycardia is a relatively common arrhythmia in pediatrics and occurs in much greater rates than other arrhythmias. This rhythm should be suspected in a pediatric patient with sudden-onset symptoms of tachycardia accompanied by poor perfusion. Heart rates are typically 140–280 beats/min, with higher rates in younger children. While an electrocardiogram (ECG) is needed to truly identify this condition, in-flight this will not be available. However, high heart rates, should put this on the differential, and some attempts to improve this rhythm can be attempted with minimal harm if this is not the correct diagnosis. Asking older patients to increase vasovagal tone (such as by instructing the patient to bear down as if having a bowel movement) may help. Applying an ice pack over the eyes and nasal bridge of an infant can stimulate the diving reflex and may break this rhythm. While it may not be successful, this maneuver little risk to the patient. If this rhythm is being considered, AED pads should be applied and an IV fluid bolus should also be considered for other causes of tachycardia, including volume loss and infection [8].

Bradycardia. Bradycardia is rare in children and often is related to respiratory issues. A complete heart and lung examination should be completed upon discovering bradycardia. It is also important to note that bradycardia is relative to the age of the patient: neonatal bradycardia is classified as heart rates under 100 beats/min whereas bradycardia in a teenage would be less than 50–60 beats/min. Respiratory support should be immediately provided. If there are signs of poor perfusion despite ventilation and a heart rate of less than 60 beats/min CPR should be initiated. If this is persistent, intravenous epinephrine and atropine can be considered. AED pads should be placed immediately [8].

9.3.3 Neurologic Issues

Altered mental status. Change in mental status can have a variety of causes, including seizure, ingestion, endocrine abnormalities, trauma, or infection. Very few of these can be directly identified and treated effectively while in flight. Glucose level by finger stick and basic airway and circulatory management should be provided [20]. If ingestion is suspected, poison control can be contacted via the flight crew. Alcohol ingestion on board should result in repeat glucose checks as this can cause hypoglycemia, particularly in young children, though glucometers are typically not included on board commercial aircraft [21]. Providers should not attempt to induce vomiting as this may pose a risk to the patient's airway.

Seizures. Seizures are among the most common pediatric neurologic emergencies encountered [8]. Frequently, seizures self-resolve within 5 min and the child may be postictal for up to 30 min following the event. Respirations should be monitored closely and assistance provided if the child is not breathing adequately. If available, a finger stick should be obtained along with gaining IV access. For seizures lasting more than 5 min, administration of a benzodiazepine (if available) should be considered. Dosing for this is as follows (see Table 9.2 for weight estimations):

Diazepam—0.05–0.3 mg/kg IV or 0.5 mg/kg PR (max 20 mg)
Lorazepam—0.05–0.1 mg/kg IV or IM
Midazolam—0.05–0.1 mg/kg IV or 0.1–0.15 mg/kg IM

Stroke. Stroke is extremely rare in pediatrics and occurs at a rate of 13/100,000 per year (higher in neonates) compared to the adult rate of 175–200/100,000 per year. Symptoms can present with unilateral facial droop, limb weakness, or slurred speech, though these symptoms may be more or less subtle based on age. Management of an acute stroke is similar to adults. Because hypoglycemia can mimic stroke and is easy to reverse, a glucose level should be obtained, if possible. The patient should be monitored closely for any worsening symptoms while awaiting definitive medical care. Definite care should be obtained within 4.5 h of symptom onset if possible. Diversion should be considered if an acute stroke is suspected [22].

9.3.4 Endocrine Issues

Hypoglycemia. Hypoglycemia is particularly prevalent in neonates, especially with premature infants. This condition should be suspected in a tremulous or seizing infant. A glucose level diagnostic of hypoglycemia is based on age: In the neonate (up to 3 mos), glucose levels less than 40 mg/dL indicate hypoglycemia; otherwise, under 60 mg/dL is used as the low end of normal.

If a hypoglycemic patient is alert, feeding should be attempted. In neonates, this includes formula or breast-feeding, and in older children, juice followed by a mixed protein and carbohydrate food item. If there is concern about the patient's mental status, IV access should be obtained. Appropriate glucose dosing is based on age. High-concentration glucose is not appropriate for all ages and D50 can be caustic to vasculature in any age group. In infants (under 1 yr), D10 is used. In toddlers to school aged (1–12 yrs old), either D10 or D25 is appropriate [8].

A provider can make a solution of D25 by discarding 25 mL out of one ampule of D50, and then drawing 25 mL of normal saline (NS) or sterile water into the dextrose ampule. To make D10%, the provider can discard 40 mL out of one ampule of D50, and then draw 40 mL of NS or sterile water into the dextrose ampule.

Glucagon may also be available on a flight. This medication can also be dosed IM if IV access is not available. In children under 8 yrs old, the glucagon dose is 0.5 mg IM. In patients over 8 yrs old, the dose is 1 mg IM. Note that this medication has limited utility in young infants due to its mechanism of action. Infants under 1 have lower glycogen stores in their livers, and therefore do not release glucose as readily with glucagon administration [8].

Hyperglycemia. The incidental finding of high blood sugar may occur with a vomiting patient or a patient with changes in mental status. Glucose levels greater than 250 mg/dL can result in significant pathology. Insulin administration for children with diabetes is appropriate if a reliable guardian knows the appropriate dosing and has the medication for a child. Otherwise IV fluids with a bolus of 20 mL/kg should be given, with a repeat finger stick (if a glucometer is available) and second bolus if glucose is still elevated above 250 mg/dL [23].

9.3.5 Infectious Disease

Overall, the role of an in-flight provider is not necessarily to make a definitive diagnosis, particularly in the field of infectious diseases. Children often have high fevers from more benign sources than adults. Ibuprofen and acetaminophen should be considered for antipyretics. Many viral illnesses can have multiple symptoms including fever, cough, rhinorrhea, congestion, vomiting, diarrhea, or rash. Treatment en route is symptomatic primarily. An additional consideration is isolation. A pediatrics patient that becomes suddenly ill may be exposing other passengers to the same illness. If he or she appears unwell, an attempt to isolate the patient may be considered. This can be a particular challenge on a flight, but a mask or cloth over the face may help protect other passengers from a coughing or sneezing child [23].

9.3.6 Gastrointestinal

Most serious gastrointestinal emergencies cannot be definitively cared for aboard a commercial airliner. The most important aspects of care include repeated abdominal examinations and symptomatic improvement. Abdominal pain may indicate a surgical need or something more benign, such as constipation. Repeat exams can help indicate improvement or localization of symptoms. Resolution of symptoms with normal vital signs may point to a less severe cause that can wait for standard descent. Persistent localized pain, particularly in the right lower and less often right upper quadrants, can signify appendicitis (common in pediatrics) or cholecystitis (rare in children), and may worsen over time as inflammation progresses. Vomiting can be treated with an antiemetic. Commonly, ondansetron is used as it can be given IV or by oral dissolving tablet. These tablets can be split to give as little as 1 mg.

9.3.7 Dermatologic

Rarely does a rash require emergent care. Diphenhydramine, or a dye and color-free body cream or lotion, if available, may relieve itching. Children often develop rashes in relation to viral illness, so a history of viral symptoms should be discussed. Anaphylaxis should be considered in acute-onset urticarial rashes (see anaphylaxis management above).

Burns. Burns may occur on an aircraft, especially if hot beverages are consumed onboard. Burn assessment and management differ slightly based on age. To assess a burn, clothing must be removed from the areas of the burn in order to avoid trapping heat against the body, which may result in increased depth of injury. Cool wet cloths may be applied, but avoid ice on the burn as it can result in additional tissue injury. Burn assessment includes estimating the percentage of the body burned. In all patients (adult and child), the patient's palm and fingers are approximately 1% of the body surface area. This can be used to estimate total surface area of burn. Use caution, as this may underestimate the extent of the burn in children and overestimate in adult women [24]. Fluid replacement is crucial, even more so in children than adults. While the extent of replacement is debated, it is appropriate to give a 20 cm³/kg bolus of normal saline. If landing time will be prolonged, the following formula can be used to administer appropriate fluids:

Estimated fluid resuscitation = 4 mL × weight (kg) × total body surface area of burn.

Half of this volume is given over the first 8 h in addition to maintenance fluids, and the remainder over the following 16 h.

Indications for consideration of flight diversion include:

- >10% total body surface area burn
- Face, hand, feet, or genital burns
- Burns crossing joint line
- Any full-thickness burns
- Inhalation or chemical burns
- Electrical burns

With large burns in young children, glucose should also be monitored due to drops from increased energy requirements in burn patients [9].

9.3.8   Trauma

Major trauma is unlikely to occur on a flight, but minor trauma may occur. Children may not be required to have their own seat (more often on domestic flights) if they are under 2 yrs of age. This means that they are unrestrained and more prone to injury during turbulent conditions [1]. Control of bleeding is crucial. Immobilization of a presumed fracture or painful limb can be achieved via an improvised splint or sling made with any firm item and cloth. A rolled magazine works well for support. Children should have their heart rate and perfusion monitored closely for signs of shock. This is due to the low reliability of a blood pressure cuff and late finding of low blood pressure with pediatric hypovolemia [8].

A relatively common pediatric injury is nursemaid's elbow, which is subluxation of the radial head. This occurs when a child has a pulling injury on the arm. It often occurs when a parent lifts a child by his or her hands, the child suddenly drops down while holding a hand or railing, or swinging a child. The history is crucial in the diagnosis of this injury. The child will usually refuse to use the arm. When this injury is suspected, treatment can be performed by hyperpronating the arm or supinating the arm with flexion. If done with a hand on the elbow, a pop may be felt when the radial head is returned to position, and within 10–15 min, the child will begin to use the arm without hesitation [23].

References

1. Alves PM, Nerwich N, Rotta AT. In-flight injuries involving children on commercial airline flights. Pediatr Emerg Care. 2016. [Epub ahead of print].
2. Graf J, Stuben U, Pump S. In-flight medical emergencies. Dtsch Arztebl Int. 2012;109(37):591–602.
3. Peterson DC, Martin-Gill C, Guyette FX, et al. Outcomes of medical emergencies on commercial airline flights. N Engl J Med. 2013;68(22):2075–83.
4. Weiner GM. Textbook of neonatal resuscitation (NRP). 7th ed. Itasca, IL: American Academy of Pediatrics and American Heart Association; 2016.
5. Butterfield J, Covey MJ. Practical epigram of the APGAR score (letter). JAMA. 1962;181:143.
6. Laptook AR, Shankaran S, Ambalayanan N, et al. Outcome of term infants using APGAR scores at 10 minutes following hypoxic-ischemic encephalopathy. Pediatrics. 2009;24(6):1619–26.
7. Rohana J, Khairina W, Boo NY, Shareena I. Reducing hypothermia in preterm infants with polyethylene wrap. Pediatr Int. 2011;53(4):468–74.
8. American Heart Association. Pediatric Advanced Life Support (PALS) Provider Manual. American Heart Association. 2016.
9. Palmieri TL. Pediatric burn resuscitation. Crit Care Clin. 2016;32(4):547–59.
10. Newman KB, Milne S, Hamilton C, Hall K. A comparison of albuterol administered by metered-dose inhaler and spacer with albuterol by nebulizer in adults presenting to an urban emergency department with acute asthma. Chest. 2002;121:1036–41.
11. Rachelefsky GS, Rohr AS, Wo J, et al. Use of a tube spacer to improve the efficacy of a metered-dose inhaler in asthmatic children. Am J Dis Child. 1986;140(11):1191–3.
12. Bush A, Saglani S. Management of severe asthma in children. Lancet. 2010;376:814–25.
13. Chipps BE. Update in Pediatric anaphylaxis: a systematic review. Clin Pediatr. 2013;52(5):451–61.
14. Choi J, Lee GL. Common pediatric respiratory emergencies. Emerg Med Clin N Am. 2012;30(2):529–63.
15. Berdan EA, Sato TT. Pediatric airway and esophageal foreign bodies. Surg Clin N Am. 2017;97(1):85–91.
16. Chillag S, Kreig J, Bhargava R. The Heimlich Maneuver: breaking down the complications. South Med J. 2010;103(2):147–50.
17. American National Red Cross. Basic life support for healthcare providers. Washington, DC: The American National Red Cross; 2015.
18. MacDuff A, Arnold A, Harvey J. Management of spontaneous pneumothorax: British Thoracic Society pleural disease guideline 2010. Thorax. 2010;65:ii18–31.
19. Friedman KG, Kane DA, Rathod RH, et al. Management of pediatric chest pain using a standardized assessment and management plan. Pediatrics. 2011;128(2):239–45.
20. Avner JR. Altered states of consciousness. Pediatr Rev. 2006;27(9):331–8.

21. Ravar P, Ratnapalan S. Pediatric ingestions of household products containing ethanol: a review. Clin Pediatr. 2013;52(3):203–9.
22. Rivkin MJ, Bernard TJ, Dowling MM, et al. Pediatr Neurol. 2016;56:8–17.
23. Johns Hopkins Hospital, Laubisch J, Engorn B. The Harriet Lane handbook: Edition 20. Philadelphia: Elsevier Health Services; 2014.
24. Rhodes J, Clay C, Phillips M. The surface area of the hand and the palm for estimating percentage of total body surface area: results of a meta-analysis. Br J Dermatol. 2013;169(1):76–84.

Obstetrics and Gynecology Considerations

10

Sarah K. Sommerkamp, Jason M. Franasiak, Sarah B. Dubbs, and Priya Kuppusamy

10.1 Introduction

During flights, medical emergencies involving pregnant women are unequivocally stressful events. A traveling physician can prepare for this scenario by understanding the pathophysiologic changes that occur 35,000 ft in the air, appreciating the various diseases that could manifest under these conditions, and anticipating the processes and complications of labor and delivery. With this background knowledge, one can feel prepared for the worst-case scenario when a flight attendant makes the dreaded announcement: "Are there any medical personnel on board?"

Guidelines regarding travel by pregnant women vary between airlines and depend on factors such as the estimated due date and whether the trip is domestic or international. Some airlines require a pregnant woman to present written approval from her obstetrician prior to boarding the flight. The American College of

S. K. Sommerkamp, M.D., R.D.M.S. (✉)
University of Maryland Midtown Campus, Baltimore, MD, USA

Department of Emergency Medicine, University of Maryland School of Medicine, Baltimore, MD, USA
e-mail: ssommerkamp@em.umaryland.edu

J. M. Franasiak, M.D., F.A.C.O.G., H.C.L.D. / A.L.D. (A.B.B.)
Reproductive Medicine Associates of New Jersey, Sidney Kimmel Medical College—Thomas Jefferson University, Philadelphia, PA, USA
e-mail: jfranasiak@rmanj.com

S. B. Dubbs, M.D.
University of Maryland Medical Center, Baltimore, MD, USA

Department of Emergency Medicine, University of Maryland School of Medicine, Baltimore, MD, USA

P. Kuppusamy, M.D.
Department of Emergency Medicine, University of Maryland School of Medicine, Baltimore, MD, USA

© Springer International Publishing AG, part of Springer Nature 2018
J. V. Nable, W. Brady (eds.), *In-Flight Medical Emergencies*,
https://doi.org/10.1007/978-3-319-74234-2_10

Obstetricians and Gynecologists recommends that women who are past the 36th week of pregnancy refrain from flying, even in the absence of any obstetric or maternal conditions [1]. Ultimately, the choice to fly is made at the discretion of the passenger, since it is quite easy to conceal the exact stage of a pregnancy. Thus, the number of pregnant passengers who travel on flights is likely underestimated.

Medical emergencies arise during one of every 604 commercial flights [2]. Obstetrical and gynecological (OB/GYN) conditions account for less than 1% of all in-flight emergencies, but they are the reason for 18% of flight diversions. Only cardiac emergencies are a more common cause. In addition, about one-fourth of in-flight OB/GYN emergencies result in hospital admission, comparable to the rates associated with stroke and cardiac symptoms [2]. According to MedAire, which provides medical training and 24-hour telephone consultation to 136 airlines around the world, there were 259 reported OB/GYN in-flight emergencies in 2015, including 3 births and 12 women in labor, whose flights landed prior to delivery. This represents 0.67% of the 38,442 medical events handled by MedAire personnel that year.

In the absence of preexisting high-risk conditions, air travel during pregnancy is generally considered safe and presents little risk to a healthy woman and her fetus. However, pregnancy induces several anatomic and physiologic changes that must be considered in an in-flight medical emergency. As the uterus increases in size, it physically displaces other organs while pushing upward into the abdominal cavity. It also compresses the inferior vena cava, diminishing venous return to the heart, leading to a decrease in cardiac output and blood pressure and a mild increase in heart rate [3]. The enlarged uterus is also more susceptible to trauma and hemorrhage. Venous stasis in the lower limbs leads to peripheral edema and predisposes pregnant women to thrombosis [4].

Pregnant women should take routine precautions to ensure a safe trip in the air. Choosing an aisle seat makes it easier to stand and walk around since periodic ambulation is recommended to reduce the risk of venous thrombus formation. Turbulence can occur at any time, placing pregnant women at increased risk for falls; therefore, the woman should wear a seat belt at all times, positioned low, under the gravid abdomen and across the hips. Since trapped gas tends to expand at higher altitudes, pregnant women should avoid carbonated drinks as well as gas-producing food before the flight. On the other hand, drinking plenty of water will help prevent dehydration, which may cause uterine contractions [1].

Even when all the necessary precautions have been taken, in-flight emergencies still occur with very little to no warning. Healthcare providers who volunteer to respond to an emergency during flight should first find a suitable space on the aircraft, where he or she can interact with the patient. Passengers can be moved around if necessary. Two places with extra room are the first-class section, with its reclining seats, and the galley area. The galley is the best location if oxygen administration is required. The Federal Aviation Administration (FAA) requires an emergency medical kit to be kept on all aircraft with a payload capacity of 7,500 pounds or more with at least 1 flight attendant on duty. The kit must contain specific medications and equipment, including normal saline, gloves, a sphygmomanometer, intravenous line supplies, and scissors [5].

The following sections discuss specific in-flight obstetric and gynecologic emergencies: vaginal bleeding, labor and delivery, eclampsia, pulmonary embolism, and cardiac arrest.

10.2   Vaginal Bleeding in Pregnancy

Vaginal bleeding is common during pregnancy. It can be caused by something as benign as localized vaginal tissue irritation, or it could indicate a more pressing situation, such as spontaneous miscarriage or early labor, with loss of the cervical mucous plug (known as the "bloody show"). Bleeding can also herald a life-threatening process such as ectopic pregnancy, placenta previa, or placental abruption. Patients with minor vaginal bleeding are not likely to seek attention during a flight. Those with heavier bleeding or hemorrhage will probably seek help, especially if it is accompanied by pain, dizziness, or signs of a major complication.

It is unlikely that a specific diagnosis can be made during flight, unless the woman experiences a spontaneous abortion or delivers a baby. The decision regarding diversion of the plane for a pregnant woman with vaginal bleeding is, of course, complex and depends on factors such as the patient's hemodynamic stability, the amount of hemorrhage, and the likelihood that the condition will worsen for the mother and the fetus. If the mother is hypotensive or tachycardic, exhibits pallor, displays altered sensorium, or has abdominal peritoneal signs, diversion should be discussed with the flight crew and ground support. In addition, an intravenous (IV) line should be established to administer fluids and vital signs should be checked frequently, with the information being conveyed immediately to the ground transport team.

10.3   Contractions, Labor, and Delivery

Contractions. Contractions are common in late pregnancy. They can be either benign or an indication that delivery is imminent. Braxton Hicks contractions are irregular, brief episodes of discomfort that do not result in change to the cervix. True contractions, signifying the early stages of labor, are characterized by regularly spaced uterine contractions with progressively increasing intensity and decreasing intervals.

Rupture of Membranes. Leakage of fluid from the vagina is significant for several reasons. First, if the presenting part of the fetus is not fixed in the pelvis, the umbilical cord can become prolapsed and compressed. Second, labor is likely to begin soon after the membranes rupture. Finally, the risk of intrauterine infection rises if delivery is delayed after membrane rupture. If a pregnant woman suspects that her membranes have ruptured during a flight, the best course of action is to monitor her closely for contractions and to seek obstetric care as soon as reasonably possible.

Location and Positioning. The patient should be moved to an area with as much space as possible to accommodate her positioning as well as those assisting with the delivery. The aisle, entryway, and galley (or a flat-bed seat, if available) offer the best options. Makeshift privacy screens can be created with blankets and jackets. The mother should be placed in a dorsal lithotomy position in preparation for a high-risk in-flight delivery.

Assess for Crowning. If possible, and after obtaining consent, a visual inspection of the perineum should be performed. Delivery is imminent if the perineum is distended and the fetal scalp (or other presenting fetal part) is seen through the separating labia.

Instruct Assistants to Gather Supplies for Delivery. In addition to items in the emergency medical kit, several other supplies must be located and/or improvised. A responding provider will need at least 4 towels, warm water, scissors (which might be included in an enhanced emergency medical kit, nonmedical scissors can be used after being cleaned with alcohol), and shoe strings to tie the umbilical cord (some enhanced emergency medical kits contain umbilical clamps or Kelly clamps). Other passengers may have these items in their carry-on baggage.

IV Access and Oxygen. If time allows, it would be prudent to establish IV access so that the passenger can receive an infusion of fluids. The administration of supplemental oxygen should also be considered.

Uncomplicated Spontaneous Vaginal Delivery. Fortunately, most spontaneous vaginal deliveries require minimal intervention and will proceed in a predictable sequence of events. The uncomplicated spontaneous vaginal delivery begins with the fetus in a vertex position (head down), with the occiput anterior (in relation to the mother). Routine or prophylactic episiotomy is no longer recommended. The patient should be encouraged to push with contractions and to rest between them. The provider assisting with a delivery should place the palm of one hand on the infant's head to provide gentle support for its slow and controlled delivery, and should support the perineum with the other hand. Once the head is expelled, the neck should be palpated to feel for a nuchal cord. If a loop is present, it should be loosened gently and slipped over the head. If this cannot be done easily, the cord should be double clamped tied, cut in-between, proceeding quickly with the remainder of the delivery. Tight nuchal cords complicate approximately 6% of all deliveries but are not associated with worse outcomes than those without a cord loop [6].

After delivery of the head, the infant's nose and mouth should be wiped with a warm, wet cloth. Suctioning is no longer routinely indicated. The fetus will then rotate spontaneously to be transverse, so that the occiput is lateral, against one of the mother's thighs. In most cases, the shoulders are delivered spontaneously. Delivery of the shoulders can be aided by grasping the sides of the head and applying very gentle downward traction until the anterior shoulder appears beneath the pubic arch. The posterior shoulder is then delivered by gentle upward traction and the rest of the body should follow without difficulty. If needed, moderate traction in the long axis of the infant can be applied on the exposed trunk, taking care not to hook or pull on the axillae, as this can cause brachial plexus injury. Infants are extremely slippery, so one must be prepared to catch and transition the infant onto the mother's abdomen.

Traditionally, the umbilical cord is clamped and cut in the first few minutes after birth. If the kit includes surgical clamps, umbilical clamps, sterile scissors, or scalpels, they may be used to cut the cord. Two clamps are placed approximately 2 cm apart, 4–5 cm from the infant's abdomen. With the infant at or slightly below the level of the vaginal introitus, the cord is cut between the two clamps or ties. If no medical-grade clamps, scissors, or scalpels are available, strings such as shoelaces can be used to tie off the umbilical cord. In this scenario, the goal is to do no harm, so, for the infant's safety, the cord should not be cut because of the potential for inadequate closure of the umbilical stump. Definitive management of the cord can be completed when appropriate clamps are available.

A newly-born infant who is vigorous, i.e., has strong respiratory effort, good muscle tone, and a heart rate >100 beats/min, should be placed skin-to-skin on the mother's chest for warmth. Additionally, the infant should be guided to the mother's breast for latching and suckling, which will stimulate oxytocin release in the mother and thus uterine contraction and involution, preventing postpartum hemorrhage. If the infant is NOT vigorous, i.e., has poor respirations, color, or tone or has a heart rate <100 beats/min, neonatal resuscitation should be initiated immediately (see Chap. 9).

Immediately after birth, the uterus should be palpated from the exterior to assess for size and consistency and to check for an additional fetus. If it is reasonably firm and bleeding is not severe, the provider should wait passively for signs of placental detachment, which can occur as early as 1 min, but usually within 5 min after birth. Signs of placental detachment include a small gush of blood, increased firmness of the fundus, lengthening of the cord, and rise of the uterus into the abdomen. The mother should be instructed to bear down gently while the cord is held taut but without traction. Once the placenta has been expelled into the vagina, the cord can be guided gently with a twisting motion to remove it completely. Uterine massage after placental delivery, in addition to the oxytocin release from nursing, will cause contraction of the uterus. The tone of the uterus should be reevaluated frequently until the plane lands and the mother and newborn are transported to the hospital.

10.3.1 Complications

Complications of delivery include nuchal cord, umbilical cord prolapse, shoulder dystocia, breech presentation, vaginal lacerations, and postpartum hemorrhage. Management of a nuchal cord is described above. Umbilical cord prolapse may be seen or palpated on vaginal inspection. It is a true emergency, as the cord is easily compressed by the fetus. The mother should be placed in a knee-to-chest position or Trendelenburg position to relieve pressure on the prolapsed cord, followed by the insertion of a sterile gloved hand into the vagina to manually displace the presenting part off the cord. In this case, flight diversion should be discussed with the pilot and should be recommended if at all possible.

Shoulder dystocia is a serious complication of the delivery process, in which the anterior shoulder is wedged behind the pubic symphysis. The umbilical cord becomes compressed, affecting fetal circulation. Any delay in delivery of the anterior shoulder should raise suspicion for shoulder dystocia. Several maneuvers can be used in this situation. The McRoberts maneuver is the initial technique of choice because of its relative simplicity and effectiveness. In this maneuver, assistants sharply flex the mother's hips up onto her chest into an extreme lithotomy position, flattening the sacrum and shifting the pubic symphysis back to free the anterior shoulder. If this maneuver is not successful, it can be combined with suprapubic (not fundal) pressure applied with the heel of the hand to increase the likelihood of success. If the shoulder dystocia persists, other maneuvers, such as delivering the posterior shoulder first, episiotomy, or having the mother turn over on all fours, like she is about to crawl, may be attempted with the guidance of ground support.

Breech presentations are some of the most feared and high-risk deliveries, because of their rates of maternal and perinatal morbidity. Instead of a vertex lie, the fetal buttocks or legs are in the maternal pelvis. As the breech delivers, the umbilical cord becomes compressed, making delivery of the successively larger and less compressible parts even more time sensitive. The presenting parts should be allowed to deliver spontaneously with only the mother's pushing up to the level of the umbilicus. Premature traction increases the risk of head and arm entrapment, so it is best for the provider to maintain a "hands-off" approach until the umbilicus is exposed. At this point, the fetus will rotate spontaneously so that the sacrum is anterior in relation to the mother. Occasionally, the legs may need to be swept laterally to be freed completely, but again this should occur only after the umbilicus has been delivered. Next, the bony pelvis should be grasped with two hands using a warm, soaked towel. Steady, gentle, downward traction should be employed until the scapulae become visible. The fetus should then be rotated 90° to one side, exposing one of the axillae/shoulders anteriorly. This anterior arm is then easily swept out and delivered. To deliver the other arm, the fetus must be rotated manually 180° in the reverse direction. Once both arms are freed, the fetus will rotate so that the occiput is anterior. The Mauriceau maneuver is used to deliver the head. With the fetal body resting on the forearm of the provider, the index and middle fingers are placed over the maxilla to flex the head. The other hand grasps the fetal shoulders by straddling the neck, applying downward traction. Gentle suprapubic pressure should be applied by an assistant to keep the head in a flexed position (hyperextension of the neck can cause spinal cord damage). Once the suboccipital region is seen under the pubic symphysis, the body is then elevated toward the maternal abdomen to deliver the head, maintaining flexion at all times.

Vaginal lacerations are common with spontaneous vaginal deliveries. To minimize bleeding, direct pressure should be applied with a gauze dressing or cloth. The most common cause of early postpartum hemorrhage is uterine atony [7]. As previously stated, the consistency of the uterus must be monitored frequently after birth. A soft, boggy uterus is initially managed with firm massage of the uterine fundus through the abdominal wall. In the hospital setting, uterotonics are employed as well. Oxytocin (Pitocin) is the first-line drug for postpartum hemorrhage secondary to uterine atony; however, it is typically not carried even in enhanced emergency medical kits. Rarely, postpartum hemorrhage can be caused by uterine inversion. It should be suspected if the mother has severe pelvic pain with brisk bleeding and absence of a palpable uterus. The inverted uterus must be replaced manually as soon as possible, as hemorrhagic shock can ensue very quickly.

Unfortunately, labor is not the only issue that pregnant women can have in the air. Women who are pregnant can get sick with many of the other ailments touched on in this book. Pregnant women are at increased risk for pulmonary embolism (PE). The hypercoagulable state of pregnancy, stasis, and physiologic changes that occur during flight are a setup for deep-vein thrombosis in a pregnant woman. In some cases, acute PE is difficult to distinguish from the shortness of breath that many pregnant women experience because of their decreased lung capacity caused by progesterone and elevation of the diaphragm by their enlarged abdomen. Pregnancy also increases the risk of cardiomyopathy and subsequent congestive heart failure. During flight, the patient can be assessed for difficulty with breathing by measuring the respiratory rate, heart rate, and blood pressure. A physical examination should be completed, including visual inspection for accessory muscle use and auscultation of lung sounds to identify alternate diagnoses, such as wheezing in asthmatics or unilaterally decreased breath sounds representative of pneumothorax, which would require another management approach. Supplemental oxygen should be administered to patients who appear uncomfortable. The patient's respiratory status, vital sign stability, and clinical appearance should be the key factors in determining if flight diversion is warranted. Pregnant women should not be panting, diaphoretic, or appear to be in distress.

Pregnant women in the late second to third trimester are at risk of preeclampsia or eclampsia. The symptoms of preeclampsia include swelling, malaise, nausea, vomiting, epigastric or right upper quadrant pain, headache, dizziness, and hypertension. Laboratory values key to the diagnosis are not going to be available midflight. Obstetric treatment of preeclampsia varies depending on multiple factors, including gestational age and severity of symptoms. Identification of these symptoms and possible diagnosis should be communicated to the ground team and diversion should be considered. Recognition of preeclampsia is important, as it may develop into eclampsia. Eclampsia can cause seizures. A provider confronted with a seizing pregnant passenger should first control and open the airway, which can be facilitated by the jaw-thrust maneuver. Supplemental oxygen should be administered to these women. Secondly, the mother and fetus should be protected from trauma. Ideally, seizure is treated with magnesium, which probably will not be available in a flight emergency kit. Benzodiazepine is a reasonable alternative, if it is available. Finally, recommending diversion of the aircraft should be strongly considered so that the mother can be assessed adequately and the baby can be delivered emergently.

Unfortunately, a few women experience cardiac arrest during pregnancy. Cardiopulmonary resuscitation (CPR) and advanced cardiac life support for pregnant women have a few differences from the procedures used in people who are not pregnant. The most important one is that an additional person is needed to displace the uterus off the inferior vena cava and aorta. This can be done by either pulling from the patient's left or pushing from the right. It is essential to prevent downward pressure, as it can cause further compression of the venous return to the heart. Medications should be administered and electric shocks delivered in accordance with standard protocols [8]. In-flight medical kits are equipped with these drugs. The success of CPR depends on high-quality compressions. Compressions should be completed at a rate of 100–120 beats/min and there should be complete chest recoil.

Managing a pregnant patient in flight is undoubtedly a stressful situation. When possible, medical personnel on the ground should be consulted. The decision to divert the flight depends on many factors. If the mother is primigravid, and is not having regular and painful contractions, and if the flight is short, diversion might not be necessary. However, a multiparous woman having painful contractions every 5 min is likely progressing toward delivery. In this scenario, diversion should be strongly considered.

10.4 Gynecology

The gynecologic emergencies that can occur during flight include significant vaginal bleeding, acute abdomen as a result of a gynecologic condition, and complications of recent gynecologic surgery. One of the most critical decisions a volunteer healthcare provider must make is whether to recommend flight diversion for a critically ill passenger. The decision-making process must include advising the crew of possible outcomes if flight diversion is not chosen [9]. With gynecologic emergencies, hemodynamic instability resulting from vaginal or intra-abdominal bleeding is the most pressing reason for flight diversion. These conditions are discussed in the following section.

10.4.1 Female Pelvic Anatomy

To understand the management of gynecologic emergencies, it is imperative to have a working knowledge of basic anatomy and physiology, which includes developmental changes in the female reproductive system from puberty to menopause. The female reproductive anatomy is designed for conception, implantation, gestation, and delivery of offspring. Thus, something central to the assessment of a gynecologic emergency is whether it is the result of or could be complicated by pregnancy. This question should be asked by emergency volunteers in every gynecologic emergency situation.

The fundamental components of the female reproductive tract are depicted in Fig. 10.1. The ovaries, located on either side of the lower abdomen, produce a follicle that contains an oocyte. The ovulated ovum is fertilized by a spermatozoon in the fallopian tube, the conduit between the ovary and the uterus. The uterus is a muscular organ with an endometrial lining that is involved in either implantation of a pregnancy if one is present or menstruation in the absence of pregnancy. The most distal part of the uterus is the cervix, the opening between the vagina and uterus.

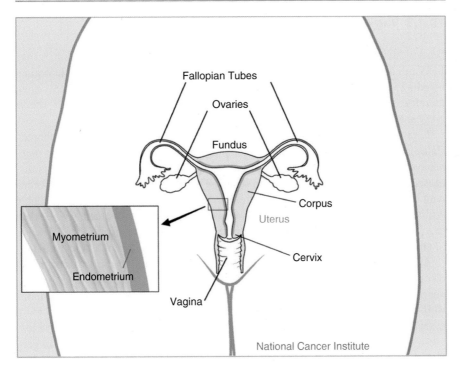

Fig. 10.1 Female reproductive tract. *Source*: National Cancer Institute—public domain

10.4.2 Female Reproductive Physiology

The hypothalamic-pituitary-ovarian axis is largely quiescent until the onset of puberty. Menarche (onset of menstruation) signifies that ovulation has occurred and, importantly, that pregnancy is possible; it typically occurs between the ages of 11 and 16 [10]. Thus, age is an important component of any assessment.

The normal menstrual cycle is between 28 and 35 days in length. An oocyte develops during the first, or follicular, phase of the cycle and is then ovulated at the middle portion of the cycle. Fertilization occurs in the distal portion of the fallopian tube and then the developing pregnancy migrates to the uterine cavity, where it implants. In the event this does not occur normally, an ectopic pregnancy may result. If no pregnancy results from the ovulated oocyte, the second, or luteal, phase of the menstrual cycle will end and menstruation will occur approximately 14 days after ovulation. Regular menstrual cycles occur in the absence of pathology until menopause, which on average occurs at age 51 (range 44–58) [11, 12]. A brief menstrual history may elucidate important clues to the cause of the patient's symptoms.

Understanding these fundamentals of female reproductive tract anatomy and physiology is important when approaching an in-flight gynecologic emergency. The subsequent sections review common gynecologic emergencies that might arise.

10.4.3 Vaginal Bleeding

Normal menstruation produces vaginal bleeding that lasts 4 days on average (range 1–8) and a total volume of about 50 mL of blood (range 20–80 mL) [13]. Vaginal bleeding indicating an emergency can occur in pregnant and nonpregnant women; therefore, if possible, it is helpful to ascertain if the woman knows if she is pregnant.

Late-term causes of pregnancy-related bleeding are covered earlier in this chapter. Causes of early bleeding included ectopic pregnancy and miscarriage. Ectopic pregnancy often presents with low abdominal pain in an emergent situation and is discussed in the acute abdomen section below. The complete evaluation of a woman with bleeding early in pregnancy requires advanced diagnostics that are not available during a flight. This scenario may require diversion so that the woman can be taken to a hospital for definitive diagnostics and treatment. Nonpregnancy-related causes of emergent vaginal bleeding include severe menorrhagia and genital tract trauma.

The initial approach should be an attempt to characterize the severity of the bleeding—its duration and volume. This characterization can be based on the number of days or hours the bleeding has been occurring and how many pads or tampons were required over a set period of time (for example, how many hours elapse before the woman needs to change a tampon or pad). Menorrhagia is defined as blood loss greater than 80 mL (challenging to quantitate in the emergent setting) [14]. In general, the need to change a pad/tampon every hour or the passage of clots more than 1 cm, which is associated with menstrual blood loss of at least 80 mL [14], is a symptom warranting concern.

The initial physical examination should focus on identifying whether the patient is hemodynamically stable and thus whether there is an urgent need for diversion. A secondary concern is identifying the cause of the bleeding in an effort to stabilize her, if possible, while diversion occurs. Vital signs should be assessed to determine if she is hypotensive and/or tachycardic. Subjective signs, such as skin pallor, are an important first step in the assessment. Further assessment of bleeding requires a pelvic examination with a speculum and imaging studies such as ultrasound, which need to be deferred until the woman can be evaluated in a hospital setting. It is important to *not* try to manually locate the source of vaginal bleeding, because some conditions, such as placenta previa, could be worsened by blind probing.

Management of a hemodynamically-unstable woman with vaginal bleeding during a flight involves supportive care and instructions to the crew that a diversion is strongly recommended. If intravenous tubing and fluids are provided in the in-flight emergency kit resuscitation, the volunteer responder can initiate their administration.

10.4.4 Abdominal Pain of Gynecologic Origin

The differential diagnosis for acute pelvic pain can be expansive. It includes pathology of gynecologic origin as well as urologic, gastrointestinal, vascular, and musculoskeletal origin. For the purpose of this section, we will focus on pelvic pain of gynecologic origin, specifically ectopic pregnancy (implantation of a pregnancy outside the uterine cavity) and ovarian torsion (twisting of the ovary on its vascular pedicle, restricting blood flow to the organ). The difference between these two might not be apparent during an in-flight emergency; however, requesting a careful menstrual history and noting a missed menstrual period should raise the possibility of pregnancy and thus ectopic pregnancy.

The priority in this circumstance is to determine if a life-threatening (or, in the case of ovarian torsion, an organ-threatening) condition exists; if so, flight diversion should be recommended to the crew. The evaluation is similar to that described above for vaginal bleeding; however, it lacks assessment of external bleeding and requires the volunteer healthcare provider to consider internal abdominal bleeding.

As mentioned above, a careful menstrual history will provide clues as to whether an ectopic pregnancy, and thus the possibility of intra-abdominal bleeding, is possible. Additionally, previous ectopic pregnancy, reproductive tract surgery, and pelvic infection all are risk factors for ectopic pregnancy [15]. A history of ovarian cysts might favor the diagnosis of ovarian torsion.

The physical examination should focus on assessment of hemodynamic instability, similar to the examination for vaginal bleeding. Gentle palpation of the abdomen to ascertain if the pain localizes to a specific quadrant of the abdomen can be helpful and also gives a sense of how much pain the woman is experiencing. If she is unable to tolerate even gentle palpation, an acute process might be occurring, so assessment in a medical facility with the capability to intervene surgically is indicated.

10.4.5 Travel After Gynecologic Surgery

Gynecologic surgery can be divided broadly into transvaginal and transabdominal procedures. Transvaginal procedures such as dilation and curettage or hysteroscopy are, in general, minor surgeries performed on an outpatient basis. Transabdominal procedures can be more complex and thus confer additional postoperative risk. All patients who have recently undergone surgery are at risk for several complications.

In general, the major concerns after gynecologic surgery are bleeding, wound infection, and thromboembolic events. Most significant bleeding would occur in the immediate postoperative period and is thus not likely during a flight. Vaginal bleeding can occur remotely from a dilation and curettage procedure and, if present, would fall into the algorithm described above.

Wound infections can occur long after surgery, possibly within a timeframe that could coincide with travel after surgery. Infections are not typically emergencies requiring diversion, other than necrotizing fasciitis, a bacterial infection that spreads quickly and can be life-threatening. This rare condition occurs after 0.18% of cesarean section deliveries [16]. Key features include tender, warm, red skin with pain out of proportion to touch, followed by a change to purple or grey with blistering and skin breakdown.

Thromboembolism is the most likely postoperative complication and the most likely to require emergent intervention and flight diversion. This condition is discussed elsewhere in this book.

Obstetric and gynecologic emergencies represent a small proportion of in-flight calls but a large number of flight diversions. A solid fund of knowledge, asking the right questions, and being prepared for emergency situations can decrease stress on the provider but, most importantly, be lifesaving for another traveler.

References

1. ACOG Committee on Obstetric Practice. ACOG Committee Opinion No. 443: air travel during pregnancy. Obstet Gynecol. 2009;114(4):954–5.
2. Peterson DC, Martin-Gill C, Guyette FX, Tobias AZ, McCarthy CE, Harrington ST, et al. Outcomes of medical emergencies on commercial airline flights. N Engl J Med. 2013;368(22):2075–83.
3. Kinsella SM, Lohmann G. Supine hypotensive syndrome. Obstet Gynecol. 1994;83(5 Pt 1):774–88.
4. James A, Committee on Practice Bulletins—Obstetrics. Practice Bulletin No. 123: thromboembolism in pregnancy. Obstet Gynecol. 2011;118(3):718–29.
5. Chandra A, Conry S. Be prepared for in-flight medical emergencies. ACEP News. August 2010. https://www.acep.org/clinical---practice-management/be-prepared-for-in-flight-medical-emergencies. Accessed 10 July 2016.
6. Henry E, Andres RL, Christensen RD. Neonatal outcomes following a tight nuchal cord. J Perinatol. 2013;33(3):231–4.
7. Bateman B, Berman M, Riley L, et al. The epidemiology of postpartum hemorrhage in a large, nationwide sample of deliveries. Anesth Analg. 2010;110(5):1368–73.
8. Jeejeebhoy FM, Zelop CM, Lipman S, et al. Cardiac arrest in pregnancy a scientific statement from the American Heart Association. Circulation. 2015;132(18):1747–73.
9. Nable JV, Tupe CL, Gehle BD, Brady WJ. In-flight medical emergencies during commercial travel. N Engl J Med. 2015;373(10):939–45.
10. Susman EJ, Houts RM, Steinberg L, Belsky J, Cauffman E, Dehart G, et al. Longitudinal development of secondary sexual characteristics in girls and boys between ages 91/2 and 151/2 years. Arch Pediatr Adolesc Med. 2010;164(2):166–73.
11. Randolph JF, Zheng H, Sowers MR, Crandall C, Crawford S, Gold EB, et al. Change in follicle-stimulating hormone and estradiol across the menopausal transition: effect of age at the final menstrual period. J Clin Endocrinol Metab. 2011;96(3):746–54.
12. Morabia A, Costanza MC. International variability in ages at menarche, first livebirth, and menopause. World Health Organization Collaborative Study of Neoplasia and Steroid Contraceptives. Am J Epidemiol. 1998;148(12):1195–205.
13. Chimbira TH, Anderson AB, A c T. Relation between measured menstrual blood loss and patient's subjective assessment of loss, duration of bleeding, number of sanitary towels used, uterine weight and endometrial surface area. Br J Obstet Gynaecol. 1980;87(7):603–9.
14. Warner PE, Critchley HOD, Lumsden MA, Campbell-Brown M, Douglas A, Murray GD. Menorrhagia I: measured blood loss, clinical features, and outcome in women with heavy periods: a survey with follow-up data. Am J Obstet Gynecol. 2004;190(5):1216–23.
15. Barnhart KT, Casanova B, Sammel MD, Timbers K, Chung K, Kulp JL. Prediction of location of a symptomatic early gestation based solely on clinical presentation. Obstet Gynecol. 2008;112(6):1319–26.
16. Sarsam SE, Elliott JP, Lam GK. Management of wound complications from cesarean delivery. Obstet Gynecol Surv. 2005;60(7):462–73.

Infectious Diseases

11

Christina L. Tupe and Tu Carol Nguyen

11.1 Introduction

Airline travel has features that are perfect for spreading infectious diseases: the proximity of passengers in a confined space for a long time and the presence of travelers from every region of the world, some of which have high incidences of specific infectious diseases. Based on a review of 34 months of data from 5 domestic and international airlines, Peterson and colleagues [1] determined that the 3 most common situations prompting calls to a medical communications center were syncope (37%), respiratory problems (12%), and gastrointestinal symptoms (10%). Any of those signs and symptoms could be associated with an infectious disease. The actual prevalence of infectious diseases among the 11,920 in-flight medical emergencies in Peterson's study group was 2.8%. Focusing on children, Moore and associates [2] found that infectious diseases, neurologic emergencies, and respiratory tract problems were the leading reasons for medical consultation among the passengers transported by one airline between 1995 and 2002.

Upper respiratory infections and influenza are spread by coughing and sneezing; therefore, droplet precautions are warranted. Most airlines recirculate 50% of cabin air, passing it through high-efficiency particulate air filters [3]. Zitter and colleagues [4] found no difference in self-reported infection rates among passengers who had traveled in aircraft with that type of filter and those on aircraft with a single-pass cabin ventilation system. The long-held assumption that passengers seated more than 2 rows in front of or behind the primary patient have

C. L. Tupe, M.D. (✉)
Emergency Medicine, Prince George's Hospital Center, Cheverly, MD, USA
e-mail: ctupe@umem.org

T. C. Nguyen, D.O.
Emergency Department, University of Maryland Prince George's Hospital Center,
Baltimore, MD, USA
e-mail: tnguyen@umem.org

© Springer International Publishing AG, part of Springer Nature 2018
J. V. Nable, W. Brady (eds.), *In-Flight Medical Emergencies*,
https://doi.org/10.1007/978-3-319-74234-2_11

a lower risk of being infected than those closer to the sick person is now being challenged [5].

The Centers for Disease Control (CDC) becomes involved in cases of infectious diseases during air travel when the organization is notified by a public health office at a county health department that a recent traveler has been diagnosed with a contagious disease. The CDC then determines if the person was contagious during the flight and, if so, then launches a search for the other passengers. The diseases most commonly investigated by the CDC are infectious tuberculosis, measles, rubella, pertussis, and meningococcal disease [6].

11.2   Patient Evaluation and Passenger Protection

During a flight, when evaluating a passenger suspected of having an infectious disease, the person should be treated as potentially contagious, especially if he or she currently has a fever or recently had a fever lasting more than 48 h. If possible, the potentially-infectious passenger should be separated from other passengers by 6 ft [5]. General infection control measures should be followed, e.g., treating body fluids as infectious, using good handwashing technique, and wearing disposable gloves. If the patient has respiratory symptoms, facemasks should be worn by the care provider, crew members who are assisting, and nearby passengers. Interactions with the patient should be brief and a limited number of other passengers and crew should interact with the person. Materials that come into contact with the symptomatic individual should be properly disposed. As appropriate, hand washing by the patient should be encouraged.

After taking appropriate steps to limit one's own exposure as well as that of the crew and other passengers, the responding provider should evaluate the passenger for airway compromise. If the patient has airway swelling, stridor, drooling, voice changes, or other significant abnormalities, recommending for flight diversion might be necessary. Patients with conditions such as croup may benefit from nebulized epinephrine, if available. When assessing the patient's breathing, the responding provider should evaluate for increased work of breathing, tachypnea, and breath sounds, using the stethoscope in the medical kit. Passengers who are wheezing could benefit from metered-dose inhalers (MDIs) or nebulizer treatments. Supplemental oxygen can also be provided.

Patients who could be septic or hypovolemic from gastrointestinal illness or insensible losses might show signs of circulatory compromise. Those who can tolerate oral fluids can be given oral rehydration fluid; for those who cannot, intravenous fluids can be started.

Infectious disease in children is also not uncommon. They are prone to conditions such as upper respiratory infections and otitis media, which can be quite painful during flight because of atmospheric changes, especially in children with poor Eustachian tube function. A nasal decongestant might provide relief to some patients [7].

11.3   Emerging Infectious Diseases

With the ease of international commercial travel, airlines have become vehicles for emerging infectious diseases. For example, during the Ebola outbreak in Africa, airlines became concerned about the transport of Ebola-infected passengers. The Ebola virus has an incubation period of 2–21 days and its symptoms are nonspecific—fever, weakness, muscle pain, headache, sore throat, vomiting, diarrhea, and bleeding. Ebola is spread through person-to-person contact and by contact with body fluids or secretions from infected people. Providers responding to a passenger who might have Ebola or similar disease should wear a facemask and gloves. Cabin crew members should be instructed to follow International Air Transport Association guidelines, which include distancing the symptomatic person from other passengers as much as possible, using a facemask, using plastic bags to dispose of tissues, storing soiled items as biohazardous material, and limiting contact with the symptomatic person, including use of gloves and hand hygiene. Ground control should be notified of the potential for passengers' exposure to an infectious agent so that authorities at the destination airport can be notified to make preparations to isolate the traveler on arrival [6].

Severe acute respiratory syndrome (SARS) and Middle East respiratory syndrome (MERS) have also emerged as life-threatening respiratory infections. These conditions are diagnostically similar to other respiratory infections, with fever and symptoms such as cough, shortness of breath, and difficulty breathing. Radiographic images obviously cannot be obtained during flight. When a passenger from an area where these conditions are endemic experiences suspicious symptoms he or she should be isolated from the other passengers as best as possible. Ground control should also be notified to facilitate isolation upon landing and access to medical treatment.

The Zika virus is a mosquito-borne flavivirus with the symptoms of fever, rash, conjunctivitis, muscle and joint pain, malaise, and headache. People can be infected with the virus through the bite of a mosquito as well as through sexual contact. The incubation period is currently unknown, but it is likely days. Pregnant women face the biggest risk from this virus, in that it has been linked to microcephaly in newborns. The treatment for Zika virus infection is typically supportive care. Because patients can present with a spectrum of nonspecific symptoms, healthcare providers should obtain a travel history. Depending on the person's symptoms, it may be difficult to distinguish Zika from other contagious infectious diseases.

11.4   CDC Reporting

The US Code of Federal Regulations requires that a report be submitted by the airline to the CDC after an encounter with a passenger exhibiting specific signs and symptoms of infectious disease [6]. The guidelines differ on domestic and international flights.

The CDC requires reporting for passengers meeting certain criteria:

1. Fever (measured at ≥100.4 F, feels warm to the touch, or gives a history of feeling feverish) accompanied by one or more of the following:
   (a) Skin rash
   (b) Difficulty breathing
   (c) Persistent cough
   (d) Decreased consciousness or confusion of recent onset
   (e) New unexplained bruising or bleeding (without previous injury)
   (f) Persistent diarrhea
   (g) Persistent vomiting (other than air sickness)
   (h) Headache with stiff neck, or
   (i) Appears obviously unwell OR
2. Fever that has persisted for more than 48 h OR
3. Symptoms or other indications of a communicable disease, as announced by the CDC through the *Federal Register*

If any reportable findings are identified, they should be communicated to the captain and ground control to facilitate appropriate isolation and medical treatment at the destination airport. As with all medical interventions, healthcare providers should document the patient interaction. In-flight care of passengers with known or suspected infectious diseases is primarily supportive, with a focus on isolation and protection of the care provider, crew, and other passengers.

11.5   International Flights

Many cases of infectious communicable diseases aboard international flights have led to contact investigations to determine the origin of the disease and to identify others who may also be at risk of infection. For example, a measles outbreak in Australia in 2010 was traced to a 12-h international flight to that country from South Africa [8]. Nine cases of measles were confirmed, 5 of them in individuals who had been on that flight. The initial ("index") case sparked a contact investigation that complied with Australian guidelines, i.e., passengers 2 rows in front of and 2 rows behind where the index case as seated were traced, as were children 2 years or younger who were on the flight. The 2-row proximity rule failed to identify other individuals who were infected, because they sat more than 2 rows away. Interestingly, two individuals who became infected on that flight were healthcare workers, who returned to their usual patient care duties after returning to Australia. The authors concluded that the 2-row rule should be reevaluated and that other strategies for contact investigation should be designed, with consideration of cabin layout, flight duration, and flight's origin and destination as well as associated costs in relation to risks and benefits.

Hertzberg and Weiss [5] calculated that passengers who sit within 2 rows of an infected individual have a 6% risk of becoming infected and those who sit beyond

2 rows have a risk of about 2%. Thus, priority should be given to individuals seated within 2 rows of the index patient, but passengers seated elsewhere should not be neglected. The authors also pointed out that exposure risk is influenced by movement about the cabin and sharing air for a long period of time. Other actions that can aid contact investigations and contain or prevent an outbreak include issuing public service announcements to educate communities about the symptoms of an infectious threat and reducing delays in the diagnosis of a communicable disease that has been brought into a community or country [8].

When an epidemic occurs, the international community often imposes restrictions on travel and escalates screening processes. In 2014, the Ebola epidemic of West Africa generated preemptive measures to ensure the safety of the public. All passengers aboard flights associated with confirmed Ebola cases in the United States were included in contact investigations and tracings [9]. In addition, states monitored individuals who had traveled from Ebola-affected countries for 21 days after their flight [10].

Conclusion

Among the multitudes of commercial airline passengers are people with infectious diseases. They pose potential risks to their fellow passengers and to the medical professionals who volunteer to help in times of emergency. Most passengers who experience acute manifestations of infectious diseases during flight require interventions at the level of supportive care until the flight lands. Medical care providers should maintain close contact with the captain so that ground resources can be mobilized if necessary, ready to receive the patient upon landing. Federal and international guidelines require the reporting of encounters with patients with specific signs and symptoms. Compliance with those guidelines can be beneficial when the need arises to launch a contact investigation involving large numbers of people. The 2-row focus of established guidelines warrants reconsideration because the characteristics of air travel (close quarters, shared air supply) extend the threat of exposure to all parts of the cabin.

References

1. Peterson DC, Martin-Gill C, Guyette FX, et al. Outcomes of medical emergencies on commercial airline flights. N Engl J Med. 2013;368(22):2075–83.
2. Moore BR, Ping JM, Claypool DW. Pediatric emergencies on a US based commercial airline. Pediatr Emerg Care. 2005;21(11):725–9.
3. Aerospace Medical Association Medical Guidelines Task Force. Medical Guidelines for Airline Travel, 2nd ed. Aviat Space Environ Med. 2003;74(5 Suppl):A1–19.
4. Zitter JN, Mazonson PD, Miller DP, et al. Aircraft cabin air recirculation and symptoms of the common cold. JAMA. 2002;288:483–6.
5. Hertzberg VS, Weiss H. On the 2-row rule for infectious disease transmission on aircraft. Ann Glob Health. 2016;82(5):819–23.
6. Centers for Disease Control and Prevention. Preventing spread of disease on commercial aircraft: guidance for cabin crew. March 21, 2017.

7. Silverman D, Gendreau M. Medical issues associated with commercial flights. Lancet. 2008;373:2067–77. https://doi.org/10.1016/S0140-6736(09)60209-9.
8. Beard F, Franklin L, Donohue S, et al. Contact tracing of in-flight measles exposures: lessons from an outbreak investigation and case series, Australia, 2010. Western Pac Surveill Response J. 2011;2(3):25–33.
9. Regan JJ, Jungerman R, Montiel SH, et al. Public health response to commercial airline travel of a person with Ebola virus infection—United States, 2014. MMWR Morb Mortal Wkly Rep. 2015;64(3):63–6.
10. Parham M, Edison L, Soetebier K, et al. Ebola active monitoring system for travelers returning from West Africa—Georgia, 2014–2015. MMWR Morb Mortal Wkly Rep. 2015;64(13):347–50.

Other Presentations

12

Christina L. Tupe and B. Barrie Bostick

12.1 Introduction

The interior of an aircraft is an austere environment for healthcare providers responding to medical emergencies. Healthcare providers who voluntarily respond to an in-flight emergency must rely on basic assessment skills and the limited supplies available on board commercial aircraft. An awareness of the conditions inherent to flight and the resources that are typically available can be of utmost importance to healthcare professionals. This chapter covers medical conditions not covered in previous chapters, such as acute urinary retention, anaphylaxis, gastrointestinal illness, toxicologic emergencies, and traumatic injuries.

12.2 Acute Urinary Retention

Acute urinary retention (AUR) is the inability to voluntarily pass urine, which can lead to abdominal discomfort and distention. Its most common cause is benign prostatic hypertrophy (BPH) in older men, with an incidence of 2.2–6.8 per 1,000 men between the ages of 40 and 79 years [1]. In a survey conducted by the Aerospace Medical Association, physicians who provided in-flight medical care reported that AUR was the cause of 7 of 622 serious medical events (an incidence of 1%) [2].

AUR can also be caused by pharmacologic reactions, neurologic impairment, infectious and inflammatory responses, and obstructive conditions. Pharmacologic reactions might be linked to anticholinergic agents such as scopolamine, which many passengers use to counter motion sickness. Those who wish to sleep during a flight might take antihistamines, which can also induce AUR. Other medications that have been linked to AUR include anti-arrhythmics, antidepressants,

C. L. Tupe, M.D. (✉) • B. B. Bostick, M.D.
Emergency Medicine, University of Maryland Upper Chesapeake Medical Center,
Bel Air, MD, USA
e-mail: ctupe@umem.org; bbostick@umem.org

© Springer International Publishing AG, part of Springer Nature 2018
J. V. Nable, W. Brady (eds.), *In-Flight Medical Emergencies*,
https://doi.org/10.1007/978-3-319-74234-2_12

antihypertensives, antiparkinsonian medications, antipsychotics, hormonal agents, muscle relaxants, sympathomimetics, nonsteroidal anti-inflammatory drugs (NSAIDS), and opiate analgesics [2]. Neurologic, infectious, and inflammatory sources of AUR are less likely as acute presentations during flight, but healthcare providers should be mindful of these possible causes and their signs and symptoms so that they can be elicited during a history taking and physical examination during flight.

Despite the cause of AUR, its acute presentation has a standard treatment: bladder decompression with a urinary catheter. Decompression relieves pain and prevents further injury to the kidneys from obstruction. In the austere environment of a plane, a urinary catheter is probably not going to be available. Some international airlines include one in their medical kit, but it is not required by the FAA. When responding to an in-flight presentation of AUR, the physician can ask a flight attendant to make an announcement, asking if one of the other passengers has a catheter. Passengers who use a urinary catheter might be carrying extras and willing to share one; if a catheter is offered under these conditions, the healthcare provider should ensure that it is sterile. When using a catheter during flight, the balloon should be filled with water instead of air, because the gas can expand 30% in volume in the low-pressure environment at altitude [3]. The patient should be monitored for hypotension caused by post-obstructive diuresis. If it occurs, peripheral line placement may become necessary for intravenous (IV) administration of fluids.

If a urinary catheter cannot be obtained, the medical care provider should alert ground control of the need for passenger treatment. It is unlikely that isolated AUR would constitute a reason for flight diversion. Ground control can organize equipment and personnel to be available at the plane's final destination. As for any medical evaluation and intervention provided during a flight, the care provider should ensure documentation, typically using forms provided by the airline.

12.3   Anaphylaxis

Anaphylaxis is an acute life-threatening emergency which without proper treatment can lead to significant morbidity and mortality. Anaphylaxis is an IgE-mediated allergic response that causes mast cells and basophils to degranulate and release histamine, tryptase, and heparin, as well as leukotrienes and cytokines. The affected person experiences an initial reaction and then, possibly, a late-phase or delayed reaction from the additional release of inflammatory mediators (sometimes referred to as a biphasic reaction). The released substances can affect the cardiovascular, respiratory, gastrointestinal, integumentary, and central nervous systems. Cardiovascular symptoms include hypotension, lightheadedness, syncope, arrhythmias, and angina. Respiratory symptoms include airway edema and bronchospasm. Gastrointestinal symptoms include nausea, vomiting, diarrhea, and abdominal cramping. Effects on the integumentary system include the classic symptoms of an allergic reaction: flushing, erythema, pruritis, urticaria, and angioedema. Central nervous system manifestations include headache, confusion, and altered mental status [4].

The clinical diagnosis of anaphylaxis can typically be made when one of the following 3 criteria is met. First, the patient has an acute cutaneous manifestation that leads to respiratory compromise or hypotension. Second, 2 or more systemic symptoms (cutaneous manifestations, respiratory compromise, or gastrointestinal symptoms) develop rapidly after exposure to an allergen. Third, the blood pressure drops after exposure to a known allergen (30% decline from baseline blood pressure) [5].

Various agents can trigger anaphylaxis; medications and foods induce particular concern in the flight environment. Foods are the most common cause of anaphylaxis and are responsible for as many as 30% of fatalities [5]. Peanut and tree nut allergies have been well publicized as causes of anaphylaxis, not just by personal exposure but also by proximity to the allergens. Anaphylaxis can also be induced by medications, particularly an antibiotic or analgesic that the affected person started to use recently.

Anaphylaxis can represent a spectrum of disease. Its severity can change very rapidly. When assessing a patient with anaphylaxis during a flight, the healthcare provider should perform a primary assessment, including assessing the patient's airway, breathing, and circulation. The airway can be affected by significant edema. The patient's voice may become hoarse. Drooling or stridor is a potential sign of an impending airway obstruction. Breathing can be affected by bronchospasm and the patient might be significantly hypotensive. Patients with severe allergic reactions can have an altered level of consciousness, and 90% of them have cutaneous manifestations [6].

The mainstay of treatment for anaphylaxis is epinephrine, which the FAA requires in the enhanced medical kits provided by airlines. On US-based airlines, epinephrine must be available in both 1:1,000 and 1:10,000 concentrations. Providers who suspect anaphylaxis in an adult should administer 0.3–0.5 mL of 1:1,000 epinephrine intramuscularly (IM) every 5 min, titrated to effect (0.01 mg/kg in pediatric patients, to a maximum of 0.3 mg). Patients who do not respond to multiple IM injections and are still hypotensive may require an epinephrine infusion. An infusion can be made during flight, while waiting for landing, by injecting 1 mg of the 1:1,000 or 1:10,000 formulation into a 1 L bag of normal saline, yielding a final concentration of 1 mcg/mL. This solution can be run wide open as a temporizing measure to maintain the patient's hemodynamics [7]. Patients should also receive an antihistamine such as diphenhydramine, which is also required in the medical kit. This medication is available in oral and IV/IM forms and should be administered depending on what the patient can tolerate. Traditionally, steroids are given to a patient in anaphylaxis. They are not required in the onboard medical kit, but they might be available from other passengers. Patients experiencing bronchospasm can receive albuterol via a meter-dosed inhaler. A peripheral IV line should be established so that IV fluids can be administered; typically 0.9% normal saline is available. The patient's vital signs, including blood pressure, should be monitored for improvement with treatment.

Flight diversion should be considered when a passenger experiences anaphylaxis, especially if the person does not respond to treatment. The healthcare provider should communicate with the crew about potential diversion, which is ultimately the decision of the captain. Patients should be monitored for the duration of the flight, because they can decompensate after initial improvement (a biphasic reaction). Anaphylaxis is a medical emergency for which responding healthcare providers with knowledge of the medications and treatment available can provide lifesaving assistance.

12.4   Gastrointestinal Illness

Gastrointestinal illness and abdominal pain are common in-flight medical emergencies. Airline travel itself can precipitate abdominal pain, for example, with changes in cabin pressure, which can cause gas expansion and make intestines bloat. Reviews of in-flight emergencies show that abdominal pain, vomiting, and diarrhea account for 15–25% of situations warranting medical attention in the air [8, 9].

In the assessment of a passenger with abdominal pain, important things to note would be a recent abdominal surgery or endoscopic procedure, recent bowel obstruction, and current use of a urinary catheter or gastrointestinal tube. Due to the decreased cabin pressure, bowel gas can expand, causing abdominal pain; the expansion has been occasionally associated with perforation. For this reason, after endoscopic or laparoscopic procedures, patients are typically instructed not to fly for a week to 14 days [10]. Just as bowel gas can expand, so can air within the balloons of gastrointestinal tubes or urinary catheters. The expansion can be controlled by replacing the air in the balloon with saline or water.

For a passenger experiencing vomiting and diarrhea, volume status is the most important thing to assess after assessing Airway-Breathing-Circulation (ABCs). It is also important to ascertain how long the patient has been sick and to ask about recent urine output. Volume status can be assessed by physical examination by checking mucous membranes, capillary refill, and heart rate. A sphygmomanometer can be used to assess blood pressure, but it may be challenging to auscultate over the sound of the jet engines.

Responding healthcare providers should consider whether the patient should be isolated to protect the other passengers. Isolation is difficult to achieve within the confines of an aircraft, but it might be possible to move the patient to a "less populated" area, such as near a lavatory, or to designate a row for the ill person to decrease the likelihood of contact with other passengers [11]. Since gastrointestinal illnesses are spread by contact, any attempts at isolation during flight could be beneficial.

Onboard medical kits typically contain an antiemetic medication, which may decrease the need for diversion [9]. Other potentially useful onboard resources include intravenous fluids and non-opioid pain medications. If the patient is hypovolemic and can tolerate oral fluids, providers should consider the creation of a rehydration solution with salt, sugar, and water (a small amount of apple juice can be added). A common recipe is 1 L of water, six tablespoons of sugar, and a half-tablespoon of salt—all of which are usually available on commercial flights.

If a provider suspects that the patient's abdominal pain is related to gaseous distension, descending to a lower altitude might be beneficial [11]. The captain and crew will make the ultimate decision, but the change can be suggested by the medical care provider. This conversation is particularly important if the patient is at risk for perforation.

A patient who is vomiting and has diarrhea or abdominal pain should be evaluated similarly to what would be done in a clinic or an emergency department. The main goals during flight are to assess volume status, attempt to keep up with fluid loss, and decrease the risk of infectivity.

12.5 Toxicology

The incidence and causes of in-flight medical emergencies related to intoxication have not been well-documented. Some studies have a distinct category for intoxication-related incidents, whereas others combine them with psychiatric and agitation scenarios. Weinlich and colleagues calculated that, although intoxication events account for 0.4% of total medical in-flight emergencies, they account for 4% of in-flight telemedicine calls [12]. Most intoxicated passengers on commercial airliners have ingested alcohol, opioids, or sedatives. Passengers who appear to be grossly intoxicated are often not permitted to board the aircraft. Also, a potentially dangerous level of alcohol intake on aircraft is relatively rare. In 2009, Girasek and Olsen published the results of their survey of 1,548 airline passengers, intended to assess in-flight alcohol consumption. Ninety-five percent of the study group reported that they would have less than 1 drink an hour during their upcoming flights [13]. The average level of consumption reported among those who said they intended to drink was about 1.6 drinks. Factors that increased the likelihood of passengers reporting they would drink were being on evening or long flights, sitting in first or business class, traveling with friends, or having already consumed alcohol on the day of the flight. Only a few passengers drink heavily while flying.

Air rage is defined as violent or disruptive behavior that affects the flight crew or passengers [14]. It has many potential associated causes, including departure delays, underlying psychiatric illness, stress, and frustration. Airline employees often attribute air rage to intoxication and sometimes the triggering event is the denial of alcohol service to a passenger. Other drugs, prescription or illegal, can also contribute to disruptive behaviors during flights [13].

A healthcare provider who volunteers to intervene in an emergency involving a potentially intoxicated passenger should begin the evaluation as in any other scenario, with an introduction, an offer to help the person, and an assessment of his or her airway, breathing, and circulation. Two likely scenarios that the provider is likely to encounter are a person being disruptive or someone who is difficult to arouse. For the disruptive person, several physical signs can suggest the intoxicating agent. Yelling with slurred speech, an ataxic gait, clumsiness, and constricted or normal pupils may indicate alcohol or benzodiazepine ingestion. Yelling with clear, pressured speech, dilated pupils, and sweaty, flushed skin are often associated with a sympathomimetic such as cocaine. For passengers who are difficult to arouse, the provider should assess if the patient is protecting his or her airway adequately. Hypoxia and hypoglycemia should also be considered and addressed. If a pulse oximeter is not available, oxygen can be administered empirically. If the onboard medical kit does not contain a glucometer, there is a high probability that another passenger on the plane will have one, though clinicians should be mindful that cleanliness of supplies cannot truly be ensured.

Treatment for intoxication will vary according to the assessment of the affected individual and the suspected agent. For the disruptive patient, the primary action is an attempt to deescalate the situation [11]. If the patient cannot be redirected and is a danger to himself or herself or other people, the next option would be restraints— physical or chemical. Most in-flight medical kits do not contain controlled substances such as benzodiazepines. However, if benzodiazepines are available, they are an option for sedation. If the person is believed to be intoxicated by alcohol or sedative medications, then the medical care provider should be careful to not oversedate, even if the passenger is yelling and aggressive during the initial evaluation [11]. When necessary, physical restraints can be fashioned from available materials. For example, a disruptive patient can be tied to a seat with neckties and other soft materials available from the crew and passengers. A physically-restrained person should be monitored for signs of hypoxia or overexertion caused by fighting against restraints, which could lead to metabolic acidosis.

In-flight medical kits carry equipment that can be used to support an obtunded person's breathing, if necessary. Vital signs should be monitored frequently and the person should be observed until he or she becomes more alert. Documentation should be completed during this observation period. Reversible causes such as hypoxia and hypoglycemia should be considered. In-flight medical kits do not routinely carry naloxone.

Overall, the number of in-flight medical emergencies caused by intoxicated passengers is low. The evaluation of these patients should be focused on their safety and the safety of others. In most cases, treatment will be largely supportive. It is up to the pilot and crew to determine if flight diversion is warranted.

12.6   Traumatic Injuries

Minor traumatic injuries are common during flights, accounting for 7% of medical incidents. Most of these injuries are caused by objects falling from luggage compartments (24%) and by hot liquid spills (24%) [15]. Passengers can also experience blunt-force injuries and lacerations resulting from turbulence [9].

When treating a passenger with any traumatic injury, the healthcare provider should be mindful of the mechanism of injury, as described by the patient, and of factors such as age, medical conditions, and use of anticoagulants. It is important to assess the patient's airway, breathing, and circulation to determine if other injuries are present. Head trauma is a common occurrence in flight. The medical care provider should obtain a history and perform a physical examination, with additional attention to a neurologic assessment. People who use anticoagulants or are intoxicated require close monitoring and reassessment. If intracranial injury is suspected, flight diversion should be strongly considered.

Passengers with abrasions and lacerations can be treated by controlling the bleeding with direct pressure and bandaging. Suture material is not available in the medical kit, but initial first-aid care is usually sufficient in the acute setting. Patients with extremity injuries should be assessed for neurovascular status. If no pulse is noted, any deformity should be reduced until a pulse is obtained. If a fracture is suspected, the limb should be splinted with materials found in the first-aid kit and placed in a non-weight-bearing position. Patients with extremity injuries and those requiring splinting should be reassessed frequently for worsening pain, which might signal early compartment syndrome or a worsening condition requiring diversion.

Scalds incurred during beverage service are very common during flights. The medical responder should note the degree and location of the burn(s) (especially to the face, hands, feet, genitalia, perineum, and major joints). Minor burns should be irrigated with clean water to remove debris and covered with bandages from the first-aid kit. An initial evaluation will usually be sufficient until the passenger can receive additional care at the plane's destination or diversion location (if warranted).

Traumatic injuries can be extremely painful. Most airlines carry non-opiate analgesics, which may not provide sufficient relief but can be given in an attempt to address the patient's pain.

Conclusion

The in-flight environment presents specific challenges to medical care providers responding to emergencies and operating in a resource-limited, confined setting. Although it is impractical to prepare for every injury and illness that might occur during a flight, an awareness of the more common conditions that can affect airline passengers is beneficial. Knowledge of the medical supplies and management options that are available on most airlines helps healthcare providers have a level of preparedness to deliver care in this truly austere environment.

References

1. Marshall JR, Haber J, Josephson EB. An evidence-based approach to acute urinary retention. Emerg Med Pract. 2014;16(1):1–20.
2. DeHart RL. Health issues of air travel. Annu Rev Public Health. 2003;24:133–51.
3. Ruskin KJ, Hernandez KA, Barash PG. Management of in-flight medical emergencies. Anesthesiology. 2008;108(4):749–55.
4. Singer E, Zodda D. Allergy and anaphylaxis: principles of acute emergency management. Emerg Med Pract. 2015;17(8):1–19.

5. Adams J. Emergency medicine: clinical essentials. Philadelphia, PA: Elsevier/Saunders; 2013.
6. Schaider J, Barkin RM, Rosen P. Rosen & Barkin's 5-minute emergency medicine consult. Philadelphia: Lippincott Williams & Wilkins; 2011.
7. Hayes B. The dirty epi drip: IV epinephrine when you need it. 2013. https://www.aliem.com/2013/dirtyepi/. Accessed 13 Oct 2016.
8. Cocks R, Liew M. Commercial aviation in-flight emergencies and the physician. Emerg Med Australas. 2007;19:1–8.
9. Peterson DC, Martin-Gill C, Guyette FX, et al. Outcomes of medical emergencies on commercial airline flights. N Engl J Med. 2013;368(22):2075–83.
10. Jagoda A, Pietrzak M. Medical emergencies in commercial air travel. Emerg Med Clin North Am. 1997;15(1):251–9.
11. Silverman D, Gendreau M. Medical issues associated with commercial flights. Lancet. 2008;373:2067–77. https://doi.org/10.1016/S0140-6736(09)60209-9.
12. Weinlich M, Nieuwkamp N, Stueben U, et al. Telemedical assistance for in-flight emergencies on intercontinental commercial aircraft. J Telemed Telecare. 2009;15(8):409–13.
13. Girasek D, Olsen C. Airline passengers' alcohol use and its safety implications. J Travel Med. 2009;16(5):311–6.
14. Kern H. The faces of air rage. FBI Law Enforcement Bulletin. 2003;72(8):6–9.
15. Qureshi A, Porter KM. Emergencies in the air. Emerg Med J. 2005;22(9):658–9.

Preflight Medical Clearance: Nonurgent Travel via Commercial Aircraft

13

William Brady, Lauren B. Brady, and Jose V. Nable

13.1 Introduction

The medical guidance provided to patients and the related determination to allow individuals to fly nonurgently in a commercial aircraft is a complex decision. The medical literature is quite robust in many areas of aviation medicine, including military applications and rotary-wing civilian aeromedical evacuations. Unfortunately, in this area of aviation medicine, the medical literature supporting this medical decision making is surprisingly limited; consequently, nonevidence-based recommendations and expert opinion are commonly encountered and frequently used by patients, travel specialists, airlines, and physicians.

It is estimated that 3 billion people fly commercially each year; on a daily basis, approximately 8 million people are flying commercially [1]. The majority of these trips occur for personal and/or leisure activities, followed by business-related excursions. Illness, whether a new event or exacerbation of existing syndrome, as well as traumatic injury can occur because of a range of issues, both related and unrelated to the travel. Medical care provided at the location of the event most often provides appropriate stabilization and treatment, allowing for ultimate discharge from inpatient management. In many such situations, the patient would like to return to their home region, not only for further medical care but also for the psychological and

W. Brady, M.D. (✉)
Department of Emergency Medicine, University of Virginia, Charlottesville, VA, USA
e-mail:wb4z@virginia.edu

L. B. Brady, B.S.Ed., M.S.Ed.
School of Medicine, University of Virginia, Charlottesville, VA, USA

J. V. Nable, M.D., M.S., N.R.P.
Department of Emergency Medicine, MedStar Georgetown University Hospital,
Georgetown University, Washington, DC, USA
e-mail: Jose.Nable@georgetown.edu

© Springer International Publishing AG, part of Springer Nature 2018
J. V. Nable, W. Brady (eds.), *In-Flight Medical Emergencies*,
https://doi.org/10.1007/978-3-319-74234-2_13

emotional need to be in a familiar location. Certain medical and traumatic events do not require significant consideration with regard to the commercial flight to the home region; non-concerning chest pain presentations, uncomplicated urinary tract infections, simple soft-tissue injuries, and basic strains and sprains are examples of such medical entities in which commercial flight is likely quite safe from a medical perspective. In other situations, commercial air travel may be delayed or not advised; illustrative medical events which can preclude an early return flight include acute myocardial infarction (AMI), pneumothorax, stroke, operative orthopedic injury, and other procedures involving gas insufflation into a body structure or cavity. Travel is usually appropriate after a period of recuperation.

Considerations which the physician must review, beyond those involving specific medical factors related to the illness or injury, include the length of the anticipated trip, the presence of medical escort during flight, and the ability of the aircraft to divert in the event of an in-flight medical emergency. Medical considerations are numerous and discussed below in this chapter. And, of course, common sense, employed by the clinician, the patient, and the airline, is a very important consideration. It must be remembered that a commercial aircraft is not a medical mission [2, 3]; thus, the expectation that trained personnel and appropriate equipment are present on such aircraft, allowing for the delivery of comprehensive medical care, is absurd.

In a related chapter in this text, entitled Chap. 14: Preflight Medical Therapies, preflight preparations are discussed; such preparations can enable a patient with illness or injury to fly with a reduced risk of adverse event occurring related to the air travel, both during flight and afterwards. Table 13.1 provides a review of the more common medical conditions, travel-related comments, and waiting days to initiate air travel.

13.2   General Considerations

Multiple significant issues must be considered in the patient with acute, chronic, or acute-on-chronic medical conditions who is considering nonurgent, commercial air travel. First of all, the "medical common sense" approach will provide the most useful information to the clinician, coupled with an awareness of the austere nature of a commercial aircraft from the medical perspective. In other words, is the patient able to tolerate physical exertion and physical stresses of travel considering basic medical principles and concepts?

The clinician must also consider the physics of commercial air travel as they relate to the patient with potential or actual medical issue, including both the lower partial pressure of oxygen at elevation, despite the pressurized cabin, and the expansion of entrapped gas as described by Boyle's law in the various body cavities. Commercial aircraft typically fly at altitudes ranging from 28,000 to 48,000 ft. Atmospheric pressure at sea level (0 ft altitude) is 760 mmHg with a marked decrease as the altitude increases, reaching an atmospheric pressure of 140 mmHg at 40,000 ft aircraft elevation. Of course, commercial aircraft cabins are pressurized with compressed atmospheric air; the cabin pressurization, however, creates an

Table 13.1 Appropriate waiting period and comments for various medical diagnoses based upon the literature, specialty and industry recommendation, and rational conjecture, assuming medical stability and ability to manage activities of daily living

Medical diagnosis	Waiting period to travel	Comment
AMI, uncomplicated, with successful PCI	**3–7 days** Post AMI	• Absence of complications • Stable without recurrence of symptoms
AMI, complicated	**14 days** After resolution of complication with stability	• Absence of complications • Stable without recurrence of symptoms
Congestive heart failure	Compensated and at baseline function	• Consider supplemental oxygen
Dysrhythmia	Resolution of dysrhythmia With sustained stability	• Consider dysrhythmia and impact on patient status
Pneumothorax, spontaneous	**7 days** Post-resolution	• Radiographic confirmation of pneumothorax • Active pleural drain with appropriate medical escort allows earlier travel if necessary or if prolonged time to resolution
Pneumothorax, traumatic	**14 days** Post-resolution	• Radiographic confirmation of pneumothorax • Active pleural drain with appropriate medical escort allows earlier travel if necessary or if prolonged time to resolution
Pneumonia	Resolution of compromise and not contagious	• Variable dependent upon pathogen and host condition • Consider supplemental oxygen
COPD	Compensated and at baseline function	• Variable dependent upon severity of COPD • Consider supplemental oxygen
Stroke, nonhemorrhagic	**3–7 days**	• Significant resolution of deficits • Absence of complications
Stroke, hemorrhagic	Case-by-case basis	• Variable dependent upon type and extent of hemorrhage
Seizure	Compensated and at baseline function	• Variable dependent upon type of seizure disorder and pattern of seizure
Abdominal or thoracic surgery, major	**7–10 days**	• Variable dependent upon type of surgical intervention
Laparotomy	**1 day**	• Also consider underlying medical condition
Colonoscopy	**1–2 days**	• Also consider underlying medical condition

(continued)

Table 13.1 (continued)

Medical diagnosis	Waiting period to travel	Comment
Orthopedic casting	**1–2 days**	• 1 day for flights <2-h duration • 2 days for flights >2-h duration
Neurosurgical	**7 days**	• Variable dependent upon type of surgical intervention • Also consider underlying medical condition
Ophthalmologic, retinal with gas insufflation	**2–6 weeks**	• Variable dependent upon type of gas insufflation
Ophthalmologic, other surgery	**7 days**	• Also consider underlying medical condition
Tuberculosis	Resolution of symptoms	• Variable dependent upon type of infection, duration of therapy, and patient response
Influenza	Resolution of symptoms	• At least 1–2 days after resolution of symptoms, likely 7 days after onset
Other infectious syndromes	Resolution of symptoms	• Variable dependent upon infectious syndrome
Pregnancy, singleton, uncomplicated, no problematic obstetrical history	No travel after **36 weeks** gestation	• Confirmation of gestational age may be required by most airlines • Consider earlier prohibition if history of premature labor
Pregnancy, multiple or complicated	No travel after **32 weeks** gestation	• Consider earlier prohibition if multiple pregnancy or complicating issue during pregnancy
Psychosis or other disturbed thought condition	Compensated and at baseline function	• Absolute contraindication to flight if decompensated psychosis or similar psychiatric syndrome • Certain psychosis patients, even if compensated and stable, may not be appropriate for flight
Decompression illness	**72 h** following treatment	• Flight prior to 72-h period after therapy requires dive medical officer evaluation

environment equivalent to only an altitude of 6,000–8,000 ft. In general, as the overall cabin pressure decreases, the partial pressure of oxygen also decreases with increasingly higher altitudes. In a commercial aircraft flying at an altitude of 40,000 ft with an equivalent cabin pressurization to 7,500 ft, cabins are only pressurized to 585 mmHg which is associated with a partial pressure of alveolar oxygen of 59 mmHg. While healthy passengers can tolerate this decrease in available oxygen without any medical consequences, patients with an acute or a chronic cardiorespiratory illness can experience some degree of compromise, including an unsafe reduction in their ability to maintain an adequate oxygenation status. With the related lower partial pressure of oxygen, patients with compromised oxygenation ability may require supplemental oxygen or may not be suitable candidates for commercial air travel. Determining which patient will develop flight-related hypoxia can be challenging; of course, the ability to do so would enable the clinician to make an informed decision.

Entrapped gas in a body cavity can also create problems during ascent or while at higher altitude. According to Boyle's law, as pressure exerted on an entrapped gas decreases, the volume of that gas will increase. This fact is of particular importance to patients flying with entrapped air or other gas collection abnormally located in a body cavity or tissue space; the primary concern, of course, is expansion of the gas during ascent. Pneumothorax is an obvious concern. Other clinical situations include pneumomediastinum, pneumoperitoneum (spontaneous and iatrogenic following surgery), pneumocephalus, otitis media, and gas installation-based interventions (e.g., gas installation in retinal detachment surgery); in addition, patients with cystic lung disease or preexisting blebs could theoretically experience an expansion and rupture of these cysts during ascent or continued presence at high altitude, creating a pneumothorax.

It must also be realized that the commercial aircraft cabin is an austere environment from the medical perspective. The ability to perform medical evaluations and care is quite limited. Flight attendants frequently have minimal medical training and onboard equipment is quite basic in most instances. There cannot be an expectation of appropriate medical care during flight, delivered by the various airlines or volunteer healthcare providers (i.e., fellow passengers who are healthcare providers and volunteer to assist). Medical escorts, healthcare providers with emergency medical capabilities, can be arranged for certain patients. Yet, only basic supportive care can be rendered by these medical escorts.

Lastly, the duration and route of the flight must be considered. Longer duration flights are associated with prolonged exposure to physiological and psychological stresses; largely, the medical common sense approach is the best guide, considering the flight's duration.

The flight's projected route is also an important issue. Transoceanic and other flights traversing less occupied areas of the globe frequently do not allow for route diversion and emergency landing. It is strongly cautioned that nonurgent commercial air travel planning should not include the ability of the aircraft to divert and land in an emergency setting. If possible, these diversions can occur based upon the considerations of the aircraft's commander, onboard volunteer healthcare provider, and ground-based medical advisor; yet, such diversions are potentially dangerous to the entire aircraft, can be extremely costly and inconvenient to the airline and passengers, and may not provide therapy in a time-appropriate fashion.

13.3   Cardiovascular

The range of cardiovascular abnormalities which will complicate the ability to fly commercially in a nonurgent manner is quite extensive; in fact, cardiovascular illness represents one of the more frequent considerations in this "fit-to-fly" evaluation. Acute coronary syndrome (ACS), congestive heart failure, and dysrhythmias, among other cardiovascular entities, are found frequently in the commercial aviation public. In fact, ACS and related complications are the leading cause of death while traveling abroad [4–12], particularly among older male individuals.

Of these three cardiovascular maladies, ACS is perhaps the most frequently encountered and most widely studied. Yet, "widely" studied must be interpreted with caution. A range of professional associations have developed guidelines addressing nonurgent, commercial air travel for patients who have experienced an ACS event; these professional entities comprise a broad range of expert bodies, including the American College of Cardiology, the American Heart Association, the Aerospace Medical Association, the Aviation Health Unit, the British Cardiovascular Society, and the Canadian Cardiovascular Society [13–16] (Tables 13.2,). While these guidelines exist, the recommendations are not supported by high-quality medical evidence, primarily because this evidence does not exist; in fact, previous literature reviews have noted that the guidelines are ambiguous and frequently based upon opinion, conjecture, and anecdote [5].

Seven studies, mainly focusing on acute myocardial infarction (AMI), make up the database for this issue [4, 6–11]. In the largest study to date [4], which included both unstable angina pectoris (USAP) and AMI, 288 patients were considered; it was noted that patients safely traveled on average 10.5 days after ACS event occurrence; USAP patients traveled earlier (8.8 days) as compared to those experiencing AMI (11.8 days) [4]. In addition to these medical studies, several specialty societies and agencies have made recommendations on the waiting period prior to travel after AMI. The various guidelines suggest a range of recommendations for the uncomplicated AMI, from as early as 3 days to as late as 8 weeks after myocardial infarction, a span of over 7 weeks. In the patient who has undergone revascularization after AMI, the recommended days to travel range from 3 days to 2 weeks—once again, a span of 1.5 weeks [4–16]. For the complicated AMI, with or without completed reperfusion, the time to travel is measured in weeks, up to 6 weeks after the event [4–16]. These recommendations are not based upon high-quality evidence; rather, retrospectively obtained data as well as nonevidence-based opinion compromise these various recommendations.

The clinician must consider several issues in the recently managed ACS patient, including the following issues:

- Type of ACS event (USAP, non-ST segment elevation myocardial infarction [NSTEMI], and ST segment elevation myocardial infarction [STEMI])
- Diagnostic-management strategies employed (risk stratification, coronary angiography, and percutaneous coronary intervention [PCI])
- The occurrence of complications (recurrent/ongoing chest discomfort, malignant dysrhythmia, cardiogenic shock, and stroke)
- The planned distance and anticipated duration of travel as well as the ability to divert for in-flight emergencies

The most opportune scenario, allowing for a short waiting period prior to travel, includes the stable NSTEMI patient who has undergone PCI and has a relatively short, non-oceanic flight planned. The opposite end of the spectrum, i.e., the

Table 13.2 Appropriate waiting period and other comments after AMI according to various specialty societies; note that days quoted are relative to the day of onset of AMI event or therapeutic intervention [12–16, 25, 37]

Recommendation source	Uncomplicated AMI	Complicated AMI	AMI s/p CABG	AMI s/p PCI	Contraindication to flight
American College of Cardiology/American Heart Association (2004/2007)	UA/NSTEMI: <14 days STEMI: >14 days	14 days Stable course	NA	<14 days Low risk category	• Angina • Dyspnea • Hypoxemia at rest • Fear of flying • Flying alone
Aerospace Medical Association (2003)	14–21 days	6 weeks	14 days	NA	• Unstable angina • Heart failure[a] • Uncontrolled hypertension • Uncontrolled arrhythmia
Canadian Cardiovascular Society (2003)	6–8 weeks, Normal/adequate stress testing	Address complications	NA	NA	• Abnormal stress testing
Aviation Health Unit, UK Civil Aviation Authority (2007)	7–10 days	4–6 weeks	10–14 days	5 days, s/p PCI	• Unstable angina • Heart failure[a] • Uncontrolled arrhythmia • Severe valve dysfunction
British Cardiovascular Society (2010)	3 days	10 days, EF >40% No CHF/inducible ischemia/arrhythmia	10 days, No complications	3 days, No complications	• Acute heart failure

AMI acute myocardial infarction, *CABG* coronary artery bypass graft, *PCI* percutaneous coronary intervention, *EF* ejection fraction, *NSTEMI* non-ST elevation myocardial infarction, *STEMI* ST elevation myocardial infarction, *UA* unstable angina
[a]Severe/decompensated

worst-case scenario likely requiring a longer waiting period, is characterized by the complicated STEMI patient who did not undergo PCI and has planned a transoceanic journey. The former case likely does not represent a challenging consideration nor is it associated with high risk; the latter case, however, has significant associated risk and represents a challenge for nonurgent repatriation via commercial air.

Considering the paucity of information, it may be more appropriate to base recommendations from a two-step perspective with (1) the initial step detailing the type of AMI, including occurrence of complications, (2) followed by the type of reperfusion therapy (PCI, fibrinolysis, and/or CABG) provided to the patient. A separation, such as this approach, would allow the physician advising the recent AMI patient how to proceed regardless of the geographic location of initial care, assuming that a basic medical facility is present.

In a general sense, the uncomplicated AMI which has been definitively managed with PCI likely can travel as early as 3–7 days postinfarction. Consideration of the distance and/or time of travel, however, must be made (relatively short travel period versus prolonged travel with transoceanic route); physiological and psychological issues can be significant in certain cases, particularly the long-distance/long-duration transoceanic route. Complicated and/or non-risk-stratified (i.e., non-reperfused, if needed) AMI scenarios likely require a longer waiting period, ranging from days to weeks; recommendations are best made on an individual basis in these more complex scenarios.

Chronic ischemic heart disease considerations will largely be driven by the patient's ability to ambulate, manage activities of daily living, and tolerate the psychologic stresses of air travel.

Regarding the other cardiovascular maladies, "medical common sense" coupled with an awareness of commercial flight issue is likely the most appropriate guide to determining the appropriateness of nonurgent commercial air travel. For the patient with compensated congestive heart failure (CHF), the clinician must consider the patient's overall condition, including exercise tolerance and respiratory status. While supplemental oxygen can be safely used on a commercial flight, the clinician must recall that such aircraft have passenger cabins pressurized to approximately 6,000–8,000 ft elevation (i.e., the aircraft is not pressurized to sea level). Regarding dysrhythmias, no specific recommendation can be made, other than basic stability issues and ability to manage one's self without advanced medical support for the duration of the flight.

13.4 Pulmonary

Of the various pulmonary disorders, most can be approached from the "medical common sense" approach. For instance, the patient with acute conditions, such as pneumonia or pulmonary embolism, or chronic ailments, including asthma, chronic obstructive pulmonary disease, and various interstitial lung diseases, must be viewed from the perspectives of tolerating the physical, physiological, and psychological stressors associated with flight. The ability to tolerate both these stressors and the lower oxygen tension during flight is the primary determinant of advising safe travel.

Pneumothorax has been the most extensively studied; unfortunately, the literature base considering pneumothorax, however, is also extremely limited. An active pneumothorax is an absolute contraindication to nonurgent, commercial air travel. A recent review of the literature explores this issue [17]. A very common question posed to the clinician advising the pneumothorax patient asks the following: When is it safe to travel via commercial aircraft in a nonurgent fashion? At this point, it is difficult to provide an evidence-based answer to this most important question. The majority of experts as well as the limited data suggest that a 14-day waiting period from the time of pneumothorax resolution is most appropriate [17–23]; other recommendations, however, suggest a considerably longer waiting period, from 3 to 6 weeks [17–23]. Importantly, the waiting period to safe air travel starts with documented resolution of the pneumothorax, determined by repeat radiography; "day 1" of the waiting period is not the day of pneumothorax occurrence. Other clinicians make a distinction in time to travel safely via aircraft between the two primary pneumothorax presentations, spontaneous and traumatic: a 7-day waiting period for the spontaneous pneumothorax and a 14-day waiting period for the traumatic pneumothorax [17] (Tables 13.3).

Two other questions are also frequently asked, addressing the type of definitive care of the pneumothorax and the requirement of medical escort during flight. There is no data, quality based or otherwise, to answer the first query, the type of definitive care (i.e., drainage) of the pneumothorax, and its impact on medical decision-making regarding appropriateness of nonurgent commercial air travel. Opinion-based thought suggests that initial pneumothorax treatment is best determined by the clinician; in most instances, the treatment does not impact the decision to nonurgently fly via commercial aircraft, assuming resolution of the pneumothorax and overall medical stability.

The decision to furnish a medical escort is not addressed in the existing medical literature; opinion-based recommendations span the spectrum, from no escort to physician escort. "Medical common sense" suggests that an appropriately trained and equipped medical escort should be considered for patients traveling with continued pneumothorax or for patients with a medical device in place (pleural catheter, chest tube, or relief valve). Until evidence is reported which can directly address this query, the most appropriate recommendation is to consider the patient's situation and duration of flight, among other factors.

In the patient with pneumothorax, the most rational approach to choosing the most appropriate time interval to nonurgent travel, based upon the limited literature base and opinion, includes the following [17]:

- Spontaneous pneumothorax: The time to travel is 7–14 days after radiographic confirmation of pneumothorax resolution.
- Traumatic pneumothorax: The time to travel is 10–14 days after radiographic confirmation of the pneumothorax resolution.
- Traveling with pleural drain in place: Patients can conceivably travel with an active pleural drain in place and accompanying medical personnel competent to operate the drain.

Table 13.3 Appropriate waiting period and other comments after pneumothorax according to various specialty societies [15, 16, 27, 38–40]

Recommendation source	Waiting period to travel [note that days quoted are relative to the day of resolution of pneumothorax]	Comments
Aerospace Medical Association	**14–21 days** After successful treatment	• "Pneumothorax is an absolute contraindication to air travel." • "Generally, it should be safe to travel by air 2 or 3 week after successful drainage of a pneumothorax."
American College of Chest Physicians	No time period noted	• No specific comments.
British Thoracic Society	Spontaneous PTX—**7 days** after radiographic resolution Traumatic PTX—**14 days** after radiographic resolution	• "Patients with a closed pneumothorax should not travel on commercial flights" except for those with a "chronic localized air collection which has been very carefully evaluated." • Patients with spontaneous pneumothorax should not fly until 7 days after radiographic resolution of pneumothorax. • Patients with traumatic pneumothorax should not fly until 14 days after radiographic resolution of pneumothorax.
International Air Transport Association	Spontaneous PTX—**7 days** after radiographic resolution Traumatic PTX—**14 days** after radiographic resolution	• Patients with spontaneous pneumothorax should not fly until 7 days after full inflation. • Patients with traumatic pneumothorax should not fly until 14 days after full inflation. • Earlier transportation with "Heimlich-type" drain and trained medical escort is acceptable.
American Medical Association	No time period noted	• Not addressed.

Chronic obstructive pulmonary disease (COPD) represents yet another challenge to the clinician regarding appropriate commercial air travel. In addition to the physical and psychological stresses of flight, the 2 issues of basic physics must be considered, particularly in those patients with significant COPD, including both the lower partial pressure of oxygen at elevation and the expansion of entrapped gas in the various body cavities [24].

The first goal is to determine if the COPD patient can tolerate the lower oxygen availability associated with flight. Determining which COPD patient will develop flight-related hypoxia can be challenging. Of course, the ability to do so would enable the clinician to make an informed decision. Depending upon the extent of anticipated flight-related hypoxia, the clinician can either advise against air travel or prescribe supplemental oxygen during the trip. Of course, the easiest approach is to consider the patient's preflight oxygenation status. If the patient is unable to maintain oxygen saturations greater than 92–94% while using supplemental oxygen at flow rates no greater than 4–6 L/min, then commercial air travel is not advised. Individual airlines have specific criteria regarding fitness to fly and oxygen saturations achievable while using supplemental oxygen. A simple mathematical calculation can also be used, employing the patient's arterial P_{O2} at sea level (or known elevation) and the expected P_{O2} in the aircraft cabin, using 8,000 ft as the maximal elevation, making the assumption that the arterial-to-alveolar oxygen ratio remains constant at any altitude [24].

Some experts recommend the hypoxic challenge test, considered the gold standard by many, which simulates the aircraft cabin environment in a laboratory setting. A mixture of oxygen-nitrogen is administered to the patient with arterial blood gas determinations. If the challenge results in an arterial P_{O2} of less than 55 mm Hg, supplemental oxygen is likely indicated during flight [25]. If the patient is unable to maintain appropriate oxygen saturations with supplemental therapy, has a calculated anticipated oxygen desaturation, or fails the hypoxic challenge test, then nonurgent commercial air travel is likely contraindicated.

The second consideration in the COPD patient occurs in the patient with significant emphysema-related blebs. As Boyle's law notes, as pressure exerted on an entrapped gas decreases, the volume of that gas will increase. This fact is of theoretical concern for the COPD-related bleb, which can experience an expansion and rupture during ascent or continued presence at high altitude, creating a pneumothorax. Some pulmonologists will advise against nonurgent commercial air travel in a COPD patient with significant blebs.

13.5   Neurologic

As is true with cardiovascular and pulmonary ailments, the literature does not provide significant guidance regarding neurologic conditions. Stroke (hemorrhagic and nonhemorrhagic), seizure disorder, and neuromuscular syndromes have minimal mention in various professional statements. First of all, "medical common sense" provides the best guide to determining safety and appropriateness of nonurgent, commercial air travel.

Regarding nonhemorrhagic stroke, no scholarly literature addressing the safety and appropriateness of nonurgent, commercial air travel is found [26].

Several aviation professional groups, however, have made recommendations. These recommendations are opinion-based with no medical resource supporting the contentions (Tables 13.4). Considering these opinion-based recommendations, two groups refrained from making a specific suggestion about time to travel; none of these documents provided references for the recommendations or provided any discussion beyond the text included in the recommendation [14–16, 27–29]. For uncomplicated stroke, specific recommendations call for "medical clearance" if traveling within 4–10 days of the event; in addition, nurse escort and supplemental oxygen are required if traveling within 2 weeks of stroke occurrence [14–16, 27–29].

Table 13.4 Appropriate waiting period and other comments after nonhemorrhagic stroke according to various specialty societies and industry [15, 16, 27–29]

Recommendation source	Time to travel after stroke [note that days quoted are relative to the day of onset of stroke event]	Comments
International Air Transport Association	**<4 days** Medical clearance required Uncomplicated—**5–14 days** Complicated—**5–14 days** RN escort required	• Nurse escort for travel between 5 and 14 days, unless "an uncomplicated recovery has been made" • Supplemental oxygen for all travel <14 days
British Airways	**3 days** Stable and recovering **Within 10 days** Medical clearance required	• "For those with cerebral artery insufficiency, hypoxia may lead to problems and supplementary oxygen may be advisable"
World Health Organization	**None noted** Case-by-case basis	• "Travel by air is normally contraindicated in … thosesuffering from … recent … stroke (elapsed time since the event depending on severity of illness & duration of travel)"
Aerospace Medical Association Medical Guidelines Task Force	**None noted** Once acute phase of recovery is over and patient is stable	• "Patients … should be observed until sufficient time has passed to assure stability of the neurological condition" • "… the risk of post-event complications, the physical & mental disability, & the decreased capacity to withstand the stresses of flight are cogent reasons not to fly" • "Once the acute phase of recovery is over and the patient is stable, travel may be reconsidered"

Notably, the various medical professional groups for stroke (i.e., the American Academy of Neurology and the American Heart Association) provided no recommendations about travel after stroke.

A summary of nonevidence-based recommendations regarding nonurgent, commercial air travel after nonhemorrhagic stroke includes the following [26]:

- Time to travel for uncomplicated stroke: While no evidence suggests that earlier travel is dangerous, prudent thought suggests a waiting period of approximately 3–7 days (i.e., have entered the convalescent phase of illness and are medically stable to return home). Of course, other medical and complicating stroke issues must also be considered.
- Complicated stroke with resolution of complication: Such a patient with resolved complication can likely travel by commercial air, as noted above regarding time to travel.

- Persistent neurologic deficit: The specific neurologic deficits will determine the appropriateness of flight, primarily focusing on medical safety, the patient's ability to ambulate, and the management of activities of daily living during flight.
- Persistent complication: The type and extent of complication (i.e., acute respiratory failure requiring endotracheal intubation will preclude commercial flight) will likely determine the appropriateness of such travel.
- Identifiable cause of the stroke: The specific cause will dictate appropriateness of air travel, based upon a consideration of the cause (i.e., left ventricular thrombus or atrial fibrillation with rapid ventricular response may preclude commercial flight).
- In-flight medical escort: It is suggested that a nurse escort is only required if the patient is unable to perform his or her in-flight activities of daily living.
- Supplemental oxygen: If respiratory insufficiency has been diagnosed or is suspected based upon established medical history, then supplemental oxygen is likely appropriate. In the absence of diagnosed respiratory compromise, little benefit of supplemental oxygen is likely encountered.

Hemorrhagic stroke, seizure disorder, and various neuromuscular conditions must be considered from the following perspectives: likelihood of flight-related injury, ability to ambulate and manage activities of daily living, and probability of needed urgent treatment during flight.

13.6   Surgical/Trauma

Post-operative patients must be considered for fitness to fly for several reasons, including general medical stability and appropriateness for the particular medical condition. In this instance, the "medical common sense" approach is most important.

Another important consideration focuses on procedural issues related largely to gas insufflation and/or accumulation. Patients who have undergone laparotomy should avoid flying for at least 24 h; more extensive abdominal surgery should consider not flying for 7–10 days postoperatively. Endoscopic procedures, such as colonoscopy, are associated with a minimum waiting period of 24–48 h post-intervention. Orthopedic trauma and procedures resulting in cast application should have waiting periods of at least 1–2 days. The duration of the flight delay ranges from 24 to 48 h, with shorter flights (less than 2-h duration) applying the 24-h delay. Longer flights likely need a 48-h waiting period. The concern in this instance is related to potential air being trapped between the cast and the immobilized extremity. Of course, if medically prudent and appropriate from an orthopedic care perspective, the cast can be bivalved to prevent uncomfortable or dangerous gas expansion. Patients who have undergone neurosurgical procedures should delay air travel for 1 week due to the possibility of entrapped, residual gas within the cranial vault. Patients status post-ophthalmologic procedures and/or penetrating eye trauma should avoid travel for a similar time period. Interventions for retinal detachment usually involve the introduction of gas by intraocular injections and can cause an increase in intraocular pressure. Air travel should not be undertaken for 2–6 weeks depending on the type of gas used in the procedure [25].

13.7   Infectious Disease

Infectious syndromes must be considered from the dual perspectives of the individual patient's medical needs and the issue of contagion. The "medical common sense" approach will assist with an analysis of the appropriateness of nonurgent commercial air travel for patients with infectious disease. Medical stability regarding the obvious issues, such as cardiovascular, respiratory, and neurologic systems, must be addressed and can certainly preclude nonurgent air travel. Common instances in which such air travel is not appropriate include the patient with bacterial meningitis, the patient with pneumonia complicated by respiratory compromise, the patient with pyelonephritis experiencing continued pain and inability to take nutrition, fluids, and medications orally, and the patient with soft-tissue infection-related sepsis. Other situations in which air travel likely is not inappropriate include uncomplicated infections such as cellulitis and cystitis, assuming that the patient has been treated with antimicrobial agents for several days.

Certain infections, while not always problematic from the medical care perspective (i.e., they do not create medical instability), can create the situation in which air travel may be uncomfortable or dangerous. Otitis media with middle-ear effusion, and sinusitis with significant congestion can create discomfort and/or tissue damage related to the inability to equalize body cavity pressures as flight elevation changes.

Equally important is the issue of contagion related to infectious disease. Communicable infectious illness may be transmitted to other travelers during air travel. Potential passengers who are either potentially or acutely ill with an infectious syndrome should delay travel until they are no longer contagious. A contagious illness should be considered at minimum a relative contraindication to nonurgent, commercial air travel. While a number of infectious illnesses have specific air travel restrictions, the more commonly encountered entities involve transmission via respiratory secretions, including tuberculosis, meningitis (caused by *Neisseria meningitides*), measles, and influenza. Each of these infectious illnesses has been documented to have spread among passengers during commercial air travel [30].

Although the risk of transmission of active tuberculosis (TB) is low, most experts advise that such patients with active illness should not travel. *Mycobacterium tuberculosis* is transmitted via airborne respiratory secretions. If travel with a potentially infectious patient has occurred, then fellow passengers should be notified of potential contagion. People known to have active TB, however, should not travel by commercial air (or any other commercial means) until they are determined to be noninfectious. Specifically, the traveler with active TB illness is defined as a patient who demonstrates acid-fast bacilli on sputum analysis, particularly with an abnormal chest radiograph demonstrating cavitation, or is found to have multidrug-resistant TB [30–32].

Meningococcal illness, specifically meningitis or disseminated meningococcal disease caused by *Neisseria meningitides*, is a contagious illness which is rapidly fatal. Illness caused by *N. meningitides* is transmitted via respiratory secretions. For this reason, any patient with known or suspected illness must be absolutely prohibited from all commercial air travel. Fellow passenger exposures requiring chemoprophylaxis include the following: household member or intimate contact traveling with the patient, traveling companion of patient, fellow passengers seated adjacent to the patient on prolonged flights (defined as longer than 6–8 h), and any passenger or flight crew member with exposure to respiratory secretions.

Measles, another infectious illness with significant contagious potential, is caused by the measles or Rubeola virus. Measles is transmitted by either direct contact with respiratory secretions or the patient with exposed secretion. The illness can also be spread via the airborne route by aerosolized respiratory secretions. Considering these two routes of contagion, patients with known or suspected measles should be absolutely prohibited from commercial air travel. Recall that patients are contagious for at least 4 days before development of the characteristic rash; the contagious period also extends for at least another 4–6 days of active illness. Fellow passengers exposed to measles should be notified and unimmunized considered for prophylactic therapy. Postexposure treatment, including either MMR (measles-mumps-rubella) vaccine (within 72 h) or immune globulin (within 6 days), can prevent active disease or reduce its severity [30, 33].

Lastly, influenza is one of several respiratory viruses with the potential for contagion in the confines of a commercial aircraft cabin. As with the other microbes discussed above, the influenza virus is disseminated via respiratory secretions, specifically large droplet secretions. The contagious period for the flu ranges from approximately 1 day prior to the onset of symptoms up to a week of active illness. As with other syndromes noted above, patients suspected of influenza infection should be prohibited from commercial travel of any sort, including via air [30, 34].

The Centers for Disease Control (CDC) has the authority to limit or prohibit travel for individuals who are potentially contagious with an infectious disease. Two conditions must be met regarding the traveler with contagious illness for such CDC-based travel enforcement to occur, including

- Intention to travel by commercial air (domestically or internationally) or travel internationally by other means
- Noncompliance with public health recommendations and mandates

For information regarding CDC's travel restrictions, the clinician is referred to the Centers for Disease Control at www.cdc.gov/quarantine/QuarantineIsolation.html.

13.8 Pregnancy

Due to the increased risk of in-flight active labor and delivery, it is prudent to prohibit nonurgent commercial air travel after the end of the 36th week in uncomplicated, singleton pregnancies. In patients with multiple (i.e., twin) pregnancy, pregnancy-related complications, or a history of premature labor, such travel may be prohibited at an earlier gestational age. In the case of multiple-pregnancy gestations, the limit for travel is generally 32 weeks. Many airlines require medical confirmation of gestational age for pregnancies beyond the second trimester; this confirmation should include the expected date of delivery and any medical details regarding the pregnancy.

13.9 Psychiatric

Psychiatric illness is a significant concern for the clinician advising the patient regarding nonurgent commercial air travel. Certain forms of psychiatric illness have a very low risk of associated in-flight adverse events though the syndrome itself can be exacerbated by such travel. Depression of many types likely will not produce problems during the flight. Patients should be made aware that the effects of travel-related stress, fatigue, delayed meals, altered circadian rhythm with sleep disturbance, disrupted medication regimen, and hypoxia can exacerbate the depression. The manic component of bipolar disorder, if severely decompensated, would be a potential threat to the patient and other passengers and therefore should represent an absolute contraindication to nonurgent commercial air travel. Psychotic illness can most certainly result in significant in-flight adverse event. Therefore, acutely disturbed or psychotic patients should not be allowed to travel via commercial aircraft. Patients with compensated psychotic disorders, such as schizophrenia, must be evaluated prior to travel to determine appropriateness of air travel. Fitness to fly is best considered on an individual basis with expert advice.

13.10 Decompression Illness

Divers who develop decompression illness (DCI) are at risk for re-exacerbating this illness as a result of Henry's law, which asserts that the amount of gas dissolved in a liquid is directly proportional to the partial pressure of that gas. There is unfortunately a lack of published studies to develop evidence-based guidelines on determining an appropriate surface time interval before flight. According to Undersea and Hyperbarics Medical Society guidelines, patients who have undergone successful recompression treatment after DCI should wait a minimum of 72 h before flying, so long as they are experiencing no residual signs or symptoms. Otherwise, a trained diving medical officer should clear such patients prior to flight [35]. Diving safety organizations such as the Divers Alert Network also provide real-time advice to divers for medical clearance for flight [36].

References

1. Press Release: International Air Transport Association Facts and Figures. www.iata.org/press-room/pr/Pages/2013-12-30-01.aspx. Accessed 2 Feb 2017.
2. Nable JV, Tupe CL, Gehle BD, Brady WJ. In-flight medical emergencies during commercial travel. New Engl J Med. 2015;373:939–45.
3. Brady WJ, Nable JV, Gehle B. In-flight medical emergencies during commercial travel. New Engl J Med. accepted for publication/publication pending.
4. Pearce E, Haffner F, Brady LB, Sochor M, Duchateau FX, O'Connor RE, Verner L, Brady WJ. Non-urgent commercial air travel after acute coronary syndrome: a review of 288 patient events. Air Med J. 2014;33:222–30.
5. Wang W, Brady WJ, O'Connor RE, et al. Non-urgent commercial air travel following acute myocardial infarction – a review of the literature and commentary on the recommendations. Air Med J. 2012;31:231–7.
6. Essebag V, Lutchmedial S, Churchill-Smith M. Safety of long distance aeromedical transport of the cardiac patient: a retrospective study. Aviat Space Environ Med. 2001;72:182–6.
7. Cox GR, Peterson J, Bouchel L, Delmas JJ. Safety of commercial air travel following myocardial infarction. Aviat Space Environ Med. 1996;67:976–82.
8. Zahger D, Leibowitz D, Tabb IK, Weiss AT. Long-distance air travel soon after an acute coronary syndrome: a prospective evaluation of a triage protocol. Am Heart J. 2000;140(2):241.
9. Roby H, Lee A, Hopkins A. Safety of air travel following acute myocardial infarction. Aviat Space Environ Med. 2002;73:91–6.
10. Thomas MD, Hinds R, Walker C, Morgan F, Mason P, Hildick-Smith D. Safety of aeromedical repatriation after myocardial infarction: a retrospective study. Heart. 2006;92:1864–5.
11. Seidelin JB, Bruun NE, Nielsen H. Aeromedical transport after acute myocardial infarction. J Travel Med. 2009;16:96–100.
12. Smith D, Toff W, Joy M, Dowdall N, Johnston R, Clark L, Gibbs S, Boon N, Hackett D, Aps C, Anderson M, Cleland J. Fitness to fly for passengers with cardiovascular disease. Heart. 2010;96(Suppl 2):ii1–16.
13. American College of Cardiology; American Heart Association Task Force on Practice Guidelines. 2007 focused update of the ACC/AHA/SCAI 2005 guideline update for percutaneous intervention: a report of the American College of Cardiology/American Heart Association Task Force on Practice Guidelines. Catheter Cardiovasc Interv. 2008;71:E1–40.
14. UK Civil Aviation Authority. Assessing fitness to fly: guidelines for medical professionals from the Aviation Health Unit. Holborn: UK Civil Aviation Authority; 2007.
15. Aerospace Medical Association Medical Guidelines Task Force. Medical guidelines for airline travel. 2nd ed. Aviat Space Environ Med. 2003;74:A1–19.
16. Aerospace Medical Association, Air Transport Medicine Committee, Alexandria, Va. Medical guidelines for air travel. Aviat Space Environ Med. 1996;67:B1–16.
17. Bunch A, Duchateau FX, Verner L, Truwit J, O'Connor R, Brady W. Commercial air travel after pneumothorax: a review of the literature. Air Med J. 2013;32:268–74.
18. Tam A, Singh P, Ensor JE, et al. Air travel after biopsy-related pneumothorax: is it safe to fly? J Vasc Interv Radiol. 2011;22:595–602.
19. Cheatham ML, Safcsak K. Air travel following traumatic pneumothorax: when is it safe? Am Surg. 1999;62:1160–4.
20. Taveira-DaSilva AM, Burstein D, Hathaway OM, et al. Pneumothorax after air travel in lymphangioleiomyomatosis, idiopathic pulmonary fibrosis, and sarcoidosis. Chest. 2009;136:665–70.
21. Duchateau FX, Legrand JM, Verner L, Brady WJ. Commercial aircraft repatriation of patients with pneumothorax. Air Med J. 2013;32(4):200–2.
22. Stonehill RB, Fess SW. Commercial air transportation of a patient recovering from pneumothorax. Chest. 1973;63:300.
23. Currie GP, Kennedy AM, Paterson E, Watt SJ. A chronic pneumothorax and fitness to fly. Thorax. 2007;62:187–9.

24. Johnson AO. Chronic obstructive pulmonary disease-11: fitness to fly with COPD. Thorax. 2003;58:729–32.
25. Aviation Health Unit. Assessing fitness to fly. Aviation Health Unit, United Kingdom Civil Aviation Authority; 2012.
26. Barros A, Duchateau FX, Huff JS, Verner L, O'Connor RE, Brady WJ. Non-urgent commercial air travel after non-hemorrhagic cerebrovascular accident. Air Med J. 2014;33:106–8.
27. International Air Transport Association. Medical manual. Montreal, Quebec: 2013. http://www.iata.org/whatwedo/safety/health/Documents/medical-manual-2013.pdf. Accessed 24 Feb 2017.
28. British Airways Health Services. Your patient and air travel: a guide to physicians. http://www.britishairways.com/health/docs/before/airtravel_guide.pdf. Accessed 24 Feb 2017.
29. World Health Organization. International travel and health: contraindications to air travel. http://www.who.int/ith/mode_of_travel/contraindications/en/index.html. Accessed 24 Feb 2017.
30. Illig PA, Marienau KJ, Kozarsky PE. Traveler's Health – air travel. Centers for Disease Control. wwwnc.cdc.gov/travel/yellowbook/2016. Accessed 1 Feb 2017.
31. Marienau KJ, Cramer EH, Coleman MS, Marano N, Cetron MS. Flight related tuberculosis contact investigations in the United States: comparative risk and economic analysis of alternate protocols. Travel Med Infect Dis. 2014;12:54–62. 2013;11:81–9
32. World Health Organization. Tuberculosis and air travel: guidelines for prevention and control. 3rd ed. Geneva: World Health Organization; 2008. http://whqlibdoc.who.int/publications/2008/9789241547505_eng.pdf?ua=1
33. Nelson K, Marienau K, Schembri C, Redd S. Measles transmission during air travel, United States, December 1, 2008–December 31, 2011. Travel Med Infect Dis. 2013;11(2):81–9.
34. Neatherlin J, Cramer EH, Dubray C, Marienau KJ, Russell M, Sun H, et al. Influenza A(H1N1) pdm09 during air travel. Travel Med Infect Dis. 2013;11:110–8.
35. Undersea and Hyperbaric Medical Society. UHMS best practice guidelines. UHMS. 2011. https://www.uhms.org/images/DCS-AGE-Committee/dcsandage_prevandmgt_uhms-fi.pdf.
36. Vann RD, Denoble P, Emmerman MN, Corson KS. Flying after diving and decompression sickness. Aviat Space Environ Med. 1993;64(9 Pt 1):801–7.
37. Ross D, Essebag V, Sestier F, Soder C, Thibeault C, Tyrrell M, Wielgosz A, Canadian Cardiovascular Society Consensus Conference. Assessment of the cardiac patient for fitness to fly: flying subgroup executive summary. Can J Cardiol. 2004;20:1321–3.
38. Baumann MH, Strange C, Heffner JE, et al. Management of spontaneous pneumothorax: an American College of Chest Physicians Delphi consensus statement. Chest. 2001;119:590–602.
39. Ahmedzai S, Balfour-Lynn IM, Bewick T, et al. Managing passengers with stable respiratory disease planning air travel: British Thoracic Society recommendations. Thorax. 2011;66(Suppl 1):i1–30.
40. H-45.979 Air Travel Safety. Policy. American Medical Association. Accessed 21 June 2012.

Preflight Therapies to Minimize Medical Risk Associated with Commercial Air Travel

14

Sara F. Sutherland and Robert E. O'Connor

14.1 Introduction

In order to protect the safety of passengers, airlines can refuse to allow passengers with medical conditions to board a flight if airline personnel believe that there is a risk for deterioration during the flight. Passengers who pose a hazard to other passengers may also be refused access. Airlines may require a physician to provide medical clearance if they suspect that a passenger is suffering from a condition that would be considered a potential hazard to the safety of the aircraft or adversely affect the welfare and comfort of the other passengers and/or crew. In addition, patients with a variety of medical disorders may be placed at greater risk of adverse health consequences unless preexisting conditions are stabilized prior to departure [1]. The purpose of this chapter is to describe conditions that may place the patient at additional risk during flight and outline steps to mitigate these risks.

14.2 Considerations of Physiological and Psychological Stress Related to Air Travel

While commercial aircraft are safe and reasonably comfortable, all flights impose some level of stress on passengers. Passengers must be able to walk relatively long distances, carry luggage, sit upright, and navigate the aircraft cabin while boarding, flying, and disembarking. Many passengers sit in small cramped spaces, which not only are uncomfortable but may also limit the ability to ambulate at regular intervals.

Most commercial aircraft cabins are pressurized to the equivalent of 6,000–8,000 ft above sea level during flight. To most travelers, the reduced cabin pressure compared

S. F. Sutherland, M.D., M.B.A. • R. E. O'Connor, M.D., M.P.H. (✉)
University of Virginia School of Medicine, Charlottesville, VA, USA
e-mail: sao4r@virginia.edu; reo4x@virginia.edu

© Springer International Publishing AG, part of Springer Nature 2018
J. V. Nable, W. Brady (eds.), *In-Flight Medical Emergencies*,
https://doi.org/10.1007/978-3-319-74234-2_14

to sea level goes unnoticed. Travelers with underlying medical conditions, such as heart disease or chronic obstructive pulmonary disease (COPD), may experience an exacerbation of symptoms during flight. At sea level, atmospheric pressure is approximately 760 mmHg with the partial pressure of oxygen being 160 mmHg. At 5,000 ft, atmospheric pressure is 630 mmHg with the partial pressure of oxygen being 130 mmHg. At 8,000 ft, atmospheric pressure is 560 mmHg with the partial pressure of oxygen being 120 mmHg [1]. In a person with normal respiratory physiology, at 5,000 ft the PaO_2 is approximately 75 mmHg, which corresponds to SaO_2 of 95%. In normal healthy passengers, the 30% reduction in alveolar pO_2 goes unnoticed; however, in patients with diminished pulmonary reserve, this reduction can have significant clinical effects especially in patients who have a low alveolar pO_2 at baseline. Patients who reside on the steep portion of the saturation curve can experience significant reductions in oxygen saturation with small changes in inspired oxygen.

Most commercial jet aircraft recirculate approximately 10–50% of the air from the cabin by mixing it with outside air continuously. Recirculated air passes through high-efficiency particulate air (HEPA) filters every 2–3 min to remove dust, fibers, bacteria, and other microorganisms. Air from the outside is passed through a purification system to remove particulate contamination and odor-causing compounds. The introduction of outside air at altitude makes the aircraft cabin very dry with an average of 10–20% humidity, which may cause patients to experience dryness of the eyes, mouth and throat, or airway [2].

14.3 Respiratory Disorders

A preflight evaluation is important to assess the prospective passenger's fitness to fly. Consideration of the ambient cabin pressure, duration of the flight, and destination, along with an assessment of the functional severity and reversibility of respiratory problems, should factor into medical decision making regarding suitability for flight. Patients who require supplemental oxygen at sea level will require increased supplementation during flight. Patients who easily desaturate with activity or who run lower than normal oxygen saturations at sea level will also require supplemental oxygen during flight. However, the availability and cost of supplemental oxygen vary depending on the airline; even those airlines offering oxygen will usually only offer it during flight. In addition, oxygen carried on the plane is primarily intended for use through emergency drop-down masks that are released only in the event of an in-flight emergency, such as decompression of the cabin. Otherwise, a very limited supply of oxygen is available for use by passengers.

Travelers who require oxygen continuously from point of origin to destination are best advised to make individual arrangements for continuous supplemental oxygen using portable oxygen concentrators. In general, the Federal Aviation Administration (FAA) prohibits the use of personal oxygen tanks during flight because compressed gas or liquid oxygen is defined as a hazardous material during flight. Most airlines require advance notification for the use of portable oxygen concentrators on flights and require that the device is FAA-approved. Because in-seat electrical power is unavailable on the majority of aircraft, and even if available is not guaranteed, passengers must travel with a supply of batteries that will have ample power for the full duration of the flight and all ground connections, in addition to unanticipated delays [3].

Passengers and their medical provider should consult with the air carrier in advance to determine whether a medical certificate is required and whether details on the use of oxygen need to be specified in advance. Strict instructions on the use of oxygen should include whether to be used for all or a portion of the flight, specific instructions on the maximum oxygen flow rate in liters per minute, a statement on the expected total operating time of the concentrator, and instructions to ensure that there is an adequate battery supply [3]. It should also be noted that FIO_2 will vary significantly with the respiratory rate.

Patients with a stable ground-level PaO_2 of greater than 70 mmHg, or a stable oxygen saturation of greater than 94%, should not require in-flight medical oxygen therapy. A practical fitness-to-fly test is to see if a patient can walk 50 yards at a normal pace or climb one flight of stairs without becoming severely short of breath. The hypoxia altitude simulation test (HAST) is not practical for most situations, although it is worth mentioning. This test is performed by having the patient breathe an 85% nitrogen and 15% oxygen mixture, which is intended to simulate the aircraft cabin environment at altitude. Indicators of the need for in-flight supplemental oxygen include: PaO_2 reduction to less than 55 mmHg and/or oxygen saturation reduction to less than 85% [4].

Patients with chronic respiratory disease, such as asthma and COPD, should be reminded to carry any vital medication, such as rescue inhalers and steroids, on board. Patients with chronic bronchitis and COPD are especially susceptible to significant hypoxemia during flight. Their ability to hyperventilate to compensate for hypoxemia is very limited, and clinicians should have a low threshold for recommending supplemental oxygen in these chronically-compromised patients.

Patients with active or contagious tuberculosis are unsuitable for commercial air travel until there is documented improvement with treatment to control the infection. For the safety of other passengers, patients with viral infection such as influenza should postpone air travel until clinically improved. Patients with bacterial pneumonia may travel when clinically stable, although they should be assessed for the advisability of supplemental oxygen during flight. Patients with a pneumothorax cannot travel by air due to the risk of the pneumothorax expanding during flight and possibly progressing to a tension pneumothorax. Patients who have had a pneumothorax successfully drained can travel once a normal chest radiograph has been obtained; the specific waiting period for nonurgent commercial air travel is not known. Some stable patients with a pneumothorax may safely travel with a thoracotomy catheter and a one-way Heimlich valve assembly [5]. Patients who have had uncomplicated thoracic surgery, or had drainage of the pleural effusion, should wait 1–2 weeks before traveling and be assessed for the re-accumulation of fluid and/or the presence of a pneumothorax prior to departure. Patients with interstitial lung disease, malignancy, cystic fibrosis, neuromuscular disease, and pulmonary hypertension should be assessed for the need for in-flight medical oxygen.

14.4   Venous Thromboembolic Disease

Long-distance travel is associated with a two- to four-fold increased risk of venous thromboembolic disease (VTE) and is highest in those who spend longer periods of time traveling [6–8]. The risk of VTE returns to baseline within the first 2 weeks after travel.

Virchow's triad describes 3 factors which increase the likelihood of deep-vein thrombosis (DVT): (1) a reduction in blood flow; (2) changes in blood viscosity; and (3) damage or abnormality in the vessel wall. It is unlikely the travel per se increases the risk of VTE in individuals who otherwise are not at risk. It is also unlikely the hypoxia or hyperbaric changes themselves play a role in the etiology of VTE during travel. The following have been identified as risk factors associated with travel-related VTE:

- Personal history of VTE (including travel-associated VTE)
- Recent major surgery (including hip or knee arthroplasty within 6 weeks)
- Recent trauma to the lower extremities or abdomen
- Hypercoagulable state
- Active malignancy
- Recent major surgery
- Pregnancy
- Age over 40 years
- Use of estrogen-containing oral contraceptives or other estrogen preparations
- Obesity
- Blood disorders affecting clotting tendency
- Prolonged immobilization

General measures for the prevention of travel-associated VTE have not been formally studied. However, the following are frequently suggested by experts and guideline committees for passengers during extended travel of 6 h or greater: frequent ambulation, every 1–2 h, frequent flexion and extension of the ankles and knees, and avoidance of agents that may promote immobility or dehydration, such as drugs and alcohol.

Graduated compression stockings (below the knee) that provide 15–30 mmHg of pressure at the ankle may decrease the incidence of DVT and lower leg edema associated with prolonged flights. The use of stockings appears to benefit travelers who are at high risk for VTE and has only minor benefit for patients judged to be at low risk for VTE [9].

Prolonged administration of pharmacologic agents, including aspirin, low-molecular-weight heparin (LMWH), warfarin, factor Xa inhibitors, and direct thrombin inhibitors, has proven value in the prevention of recurrent VTE following an unprovoked first event. There is very limited data, however, assessing the safety and efficacy of pharmacologic agents administered for brief periods in preventing travel-associated VTE. One randomized controlled trial comparing LMWH, aspirin, and no prophylaxis found that LMWH reduced the rate of VTE whereas aspirin had very little effect [10]. Patients who had undergone hip arthroplasty within 6 weeks of air travel who were administered warfarin or LMWH had a 1% incidence of DVT and a 1.5% incidence of bleeding. There were no cases of pulmonary embolus reported [11]. Based on limited data, it would be reasonable to recommend that low-risk patients be advised to maintain hydration and avoid immobility, and that moderate-risk patients add compression stockings to the low-risk recommendations. Patients at high risk should be assessed by their medical practitioner who may recommend LMWH in addition to the low- and moderate-risk recommendations on a case-by-case basis.

14.5 Cardiovascular Disease

Air travel exposes patients with heart disease to additional risk because of the reduced partial pressure of oxygen in the aircraft cabin. Passengers compensate for in-flight hypoxia by increasing minute ventilation, and most develop a mild tachycardia which increases myocardial oxygen demand. This increased heart rate may cause patients with cardiac disease to decompensate. Supplemental oxygen administered during flight may help prevent this. Patient should be cautioned to carry their medications on board with them and to take them at prescribed intervals.

Concerns for acute coronary syndrome (ACS) in patients traveling on commercial aircraft also include extremely limited access to medical care while in flight. One retrospective study examined the incidence of in-flight adverse events among patients who were returning home after treatment for unstable angina pectoris or acute myocardial infarction. Subjects boarded the plane an average of 10.5 days after hospital discharge and experienced approximately 1% of incidence of minor in-flight events, namely, transient SVT, anxiety, diaphoresis, and chest pain [12]. This study would indicate that cardiac patients may safely travel aboard international flights following treatment for ACS. The role of preflight provocative testing was not addressed. Patients with uncomplicated percutaneous coronary interventions are at low risk for travel by commercial airline once they remain stable and have resumed normal activities. They have no required waiting period [13].

Patients with stable congestive heart failure may safely fly; however, in-flight oxygen may be advisable for those with a New York Heart Association class III or IV CHF (i.e., those whose baseline PaO_2 is less than 70 mmHg).

Cardiac surgery, including coronary artery bypass grafting, poses no intrinsic risk to passengers aboard aircraft. These patients should be assessed for the risk of barotrauma due to decreased atmospheric pressure and should be assessed for the possibility of pneumothorax or pneumopericardium prior to travel [5]. Pacemakers and implantable defibrillators pose a low risk for travel by commercial airline once the patient has been deemed to be medically stable. It is unlikely that airline electronics or airport security devices will affect these devices, although questions related to interaction with electronics may be directed to the treating physician or the device manufacturer.

14.6   Pregnancy

Despite there being a lower pressure, the cabin environment in commercial aircraft is not viewed as being hazardous during normal pregnancy. There is an increased affinity of fetal hematocrit for oxygen; thus, the presence of a lower than normal maternal PaO_2 has very little effect on fetal PaO_2. Fetal monitoring during flight found there to be no change in fetal beat-to-beat variability, bradycardia, or tachycardia when compared to baseline. Mean fetal heart rate was within normal limits during the whole flight. Maternal heart rate and blood pressure increased, and PO_2 decreased significantly while PCO_2 remained unchanged. Respiratory rate showed a short increase during takeoff and landing but remained unchanged during the rest of the flight. No bradycardia, prolonged tachycardia, or significant loss of heart rate variability was observed [14].

Because air travel may induce motion sickness, the incidence of nausea and vomiting may be increased during flight. Antiemetic medication may be considered before travel.

Even relatively minor trauma to the abdomen during the third-trimester pregnancy may cause placental abruption. Therefore, it is important that pregnant travelers keep their seatbelts continuously fastened during flight and that the lap belt be worn properly over the pelvis or upper thighs so as not to cause injury to the abdomen should unexpected turbulence occur.

Due to compression of the gravid uterus on the interior vena cava, pregnancy poses an increased risk of DVT and lower extremity edema. Frequent ambulation, stretching, hydration, and use of constrictive support stockings may be helpful in reducing the risk of venous thromboembolism.

Approximately 90% of pregnancies that reach the third trimester go on to delivery after 37 weeks gestation. Because of this, many airlines will not allow passengers to fly beyond 36 or 37 weeks without medical certification by an obstetrician. Since the onset of labor may not be predictable, the authors believe that it is inadvisable to fly beyond 36 weeks of gestation.

Following delivery, it is generally advisable to wait for 1 or 2 weeks after birth before traveling with a newborn. While the aircraft environment poses little threat to newborns and children, this waiting period is recommended to assure that the baby is healthy and free of cardiorespiratory problems that may pose a hazard to the newborn during flight.

14.7   Behavioral Disorders

Patients with psychiatric disorders, manifesting as dangerous, aggressive, or unpredictable behavior, pose a threat to the entire aircraft and should not fly. These patients can only be cleared for flight after appropriate stabilization with medication, with consideration for anxiety and phobias that may be exacerbated by air travel. Passengers with treated psychiatric disorders often benefit from having a companion or escort to provide reassurance and assist with airport navigation. Psychiatric medications may have anticholinergic or sedative effects which impair cognitive abilities. A person suffering from substance abuse disorder should be fully detoxified prior to travel.

14.8   Fractures and Trauma

Passengers who are flying after treatment for trauma or fractures may be advised to fly business or first class to accommodate casts and the need for elevation. It is advisable for casts that had been recently applied to be bivalved prior to travel in order to accommodate swelling which can occur during flight. Following fracture treatment, it is important to determine whether or not the patient can navigate the airport, board, and deplane by themselves. If necessary, a nonmedical escort may prove essential in getting the passenger to their destination. Due to immobility and recent surgery, patients with extremity fractures are at increased risk for DVT and will likely require prophylaxis to reduce the risk of clotting.

14.9   Eyes

Air travel may pose potential problems for contact lens wearers due to dry air and for patients following surgery for retinal detachment due to low cabin pressure. Contact lens wearers and patients with dry eyes should be advised to use artificial tears. If surgery for retinal detachment involves the injection of air into the vitreous, the patient should wait for 2–6 weeks until the air is sufficiently resorbed so as not to induce elevated intraocular pressure during flight. If flight is anticipated prior to retinal detachment surgery, oil may be substituted for air as a means to reattach the retina.

14.10   Ear, Nose, and Throat

The external ear, middle ear, and sinuses must be fully patent to allow for pressure equalization during ascent and descent. The simplest means to equalize pressure is best accomplished by frequent swallowing and chewing, where the Valsalva maneuver facilitates this re-equilibration. If unable to equalize the pressure, dysbarism can occur, resulting in mild, moderate, or severe pain in the affected area. Patients with nasal congestion or allergies should consider preflight decongestants to prevent obstruction.

14.11   Decompression Illness

Decompression illness (DCI) describes a condition arising from dissolved gases coming out of solution into bubbles inside the body once depressurization occurs. DCI most commonly occurs during too rapid an ascent during underwater diving, but can also occur in other depressurization events such as air travel. DCI can produce many symptoms and its effects may vary from joint pain and rashes to paralysis and death.

Many recreational divers rely on air travel to reach their destination; flying too soon after diving may result in decompression illness. There is little in the way of scientific information to use as a basis for making recommendations about when it is safe to fly after diving. Most guidelines state that a diver making a single dive per diving day should have a minimum surface interval (i.e., presence on the earth's surface) of 12 h before ascending to altitude. Divers who make multiple dives per day or those who require decompression stops during ascent should wait for an extended surface interval beyond 12 h before ascending to altitude.

Anyone treated for DCI with recompression should have a longer surface interval. Passengers with joint pain and skin or lymphatic DCI who have completely resolved all symptoms after recompression can fly 24 h after exiting the chamber. Passengers with neurological or multisystem DCI who have complete resolution with their first treatment should not fly for 72 h after recompression.

14.12 Neurologic

Patients who are recovering from a thromboembolic stroke, who have no to minimal deficits, who have not experienced significant complications, and who are capable of managing their ADLs with no to minimal assistance can safely travel without medical escort. It is unclear if oxygen therapy is associated with any benefit in the setting of recovering stroke [15].

Conclusions

While in-flight illness or even death has occasionally been reported by the airlines, most events are not caused by airline travel, and may in fact be purely coincidental. Nonetheless, patients with a number of medical conditions described in this chapter would benefit from a thorough preflight evaluation by a physician, who would then make treatment recommendations to mitigate the risk of medical complications from air travel. Physicians who use guidelines to make treatment recommendations prior to flight are urged to tailor their treatment to the individual passenger and the situation, taking into account factors such as flight duration, flight amenities, and destination. With this in mind, even patients with chronic or acute injury and/or illness can safely travel by air.

References

1. Aerospace Medical Association, Medical Guidelines Task Force. Medical guidelines for airline travel, 2nd ed. Aviat Space Environ Med. 2003;74:A1–A19.
2. O'Donnell A, Donnini G, Nguyen VH. Air quality, ventilation, temperature, and humidity in aircraft. ASHRAE J. 1991;33:42–6.
3. International Air Transport Association. Guidance on managing medical events. Quebec: Safety and Flight Operations; 2015. ISBN:978-92-9252-698-6.
4. Dine CJ, Kreider ME. Hypoxia altitude simulation test. Chest. 2008;133(4):1002–5.

5. Bunch A, Duchateau FX, Verner L, et al. Commercial air travel after pneumothorax: a review of the literature. Air Med J. 2013;32:268–74.
6. Lapostolle F, Surget V, Borron SW, et al. Severe pulmonary embolism associated with air travel. N Engl J Med. 2001;345:779.
7. Chandra D, Parisini E, Mozaffarian D. Meta-analysis: travel and risk for venous thromboembolism. Ann Intern Med. 2009;151:180.
8. MacCallum PK, Ashby D, Hennessy EM, et al. Cumulative flying time and risk of venous thromboembolism. Br J Haematol. 2011;155:613.
9. Clarke MJ, Broderick C, Hopewell S, et al. Compression stockings for preventing deep vein thrombosis in airline passengers. Cochrane Database Syst Rev. 2016;9:CD004002.
10. Cesarone MR, Belcaro G, Nicolaides AN, et al. Venous thrombosis from air travel: the LONFLIT3 study--prevention with aspirin vs low-molecular-weight heparin (LMWH) in high-risk subjects: a randomized trial. Angiology. 2002;53:1.
11. Ball ST, Pinsorsnak P, Amstutz HC, Schmalzried TP. Extended travel after hip arthroplasty surgery. Is it safe? J Arthroplast. 2007;22:29.
12. Pearce E, Haffner F, Brady LB, Sochor M, et al. Non-urgent commercial air travel after acute coronary syndrome: a review of 288 patient events. Air Med J. 2014;33(5):222–30.
13. Wang W, Brady WJ, O'Connor RE, et al. Non-urgent commercial air travel after acute myocardial infarction a review of the literature and commentary on the recommendations. Air Med J. 2012;31:231–7.
14. Huch R, Baumann H, Fallenstein F, et al. Physiologic changes in pregnant women and their fetuses during jet air travel. Am J Obstet Gynecol. 1986;154(5):996–1000.
15. Barros A, Duchateau FX, Huff JS, Verner L, O'Connor RE, Brady WJ. Non-urgent commercial air travel after non-hemorrhagic cerebrovascular accident. Air Med J. 2014;33:106–8.

Ground-Based Medical Support

15

Christian Martin-Gill and Thomas J. Doyle

15.1 Introduction

Ground-based medical support (GBMS) is a service that is used by commercial airlines and other entities to obtain medical recommendations for in-flight medical emergencies (IMEs), or to obtain a fitness-to-fly recommendation for passengers or flight crew [1–3]. GBMS may be provided by the medical department of an airline or, more commonly, through a third-party entity that provides 24-h medical support for airlines. Examples of third-party GBMS services that have reported their experience with IMEs include the University of Pittsburgh Medical Center/STAT-MD (Pittsburgh, PA) [4, 5]; MedAire, Inc. (Phoenix, AZ) [6, 7], a company of International SOS (Singapore) [8]; and public health entities such as the Paris Emergency Medical Service (SAMU) [9]. Some airlines perform certain medical direction services within their company and contract with a third-party medical provider for other components. In the United States, most major airline companies have eliminated their internal medical departments and outsourced these services to entities that specialize in GBMS. In cases where GBMS is outsourced to an outside entity, it is commonplace for occupational health issues related to pilots and other flight crew to remain managed within an airline's medical department.

15.2 Ground-Based Medical Support Personnel

There are no current standards or regulations in place regarding the qualifications of GBMS providers. GBMS may be provided by physicians, nurses, paramedics, or other allied healthcare personnel. The services rendered through

C. Martin-Gill, M.D., M.P.H. (✉) • T. J. Doyle, M.D., M.P.H.
Department of Emergency Medicine, University of Pittsburgh School of Medicine,
Pittsburgh, PA, USA
e-mail: martingillc2@upmc.edu

© Springer International Publishing AG, part of Springer Nature 2018
J. V. Nable, W. Brady (eds.), *In-Flight Medical Emergencies*,
https://doi.org/10.1007/978-3-319-74234-2_15

GBMS are generally determined by the capabilities of the GBMS center and the requirements of the airline, as determined through direct contracts between these groups.

Most GBMS centers use a call taker to gather the initial information and route the call to the appropriate healthcare provider. A GBMS physician may be on-site at the GBMS center and directly manage all airline medical calls. Alternately, cases may be primarily managed by nonphysician healthcare providers such as nurses who consult with a physician on an as-needed basis. Physicians may be directly employed by the GBMS center or may be contracted agents from a nearby emergency department. Most large third-party GBMS centers use emergency physicians. Airlines that provide GBMS within their company commonly use physicians trained in occupational medicine or internal medicine, though some may employ emergency medicine specialists.

15.3 Types of Ground-Based Medical Services Provided

15.3.1 In-Flight Medical Emergencies

Consultation for IMEs is one of the key services provided by a GBMS center. GBMS serves as a resource for the aircraft crew and airline to address immediate medical decisions. Consultation may occur regarding what medications should be used from the aircraft's Emergency Medical Kit (EMK) or whether specific medical interventions are indicated. When an aircraft diversion is considered, GBMS may recommend to divert immediately, divert to a more suitable location, or continue toward the intended destination. Through use of GBMS, airlines aim to appropriately utilize medical resources, ensure that recommendations or treatment provided by onboard healthcare personnel are appropriate for the condition, and overall ensure that optimal care is provided for any passenger with an IME.

15.3.2 Passenger Preflight Screenings

GBMS is also often consulted to assist in determining if it is safe for a passenger to board a plane. These consultations are often made by a gate agent or customer service representative due to concern over the acute or chronic health of a potential passenger and concern about their medical deterioration during the flight. The request for a preflight screening may be triggered because a passenger makes a statement regarding a medical condition or may appear obviously ill or in distress. For patients who have had a previous medical emergency while travelling with an airline, the airline may require consultation with GBMS prior to boarding another flight. This consultation aims to ensure resolution of the prior medical emergency and determine the passenger's current fitness for air travel.

Common questions addressed during preflight screenings include the typical use of, or anticipated need for, oxygen during flight, as well as potential need for medications that the passenger usually takes [10–12]. For patients identified as having a potentially communicable disease, there may be questions regarding the risk of exposure of other passengers and any precautions that may be necessary. During these preflight screenings, GBMS may recommend that the patient be allowed to travel, recommend that additional medical assessment and care be provided prior to air travel, or recommend that the passenger not be allowed to travel until a specific medical condition is addressed. In making this recommendation, the GBMS provider focuses on ensuring the safety of the passenger, ensuring the safety of other passengers and personnel on the aircraft, and minimizing the risk of an unintended aircraft diversion for a medical emergency.

Other providers that may perform a fitness-to-fly evaluation include the passenger's own physician, or a physician at a clinic or hospital where the passenger has been evaluated for a medical event. These providers may write a "fitness-to-fly" letter that is used by the GBMS provider and/or the airline as documentation of suitability to fly. Supporting documentation may be requested by the GBMS provider when consultation by the airline follows an assessment already performed by an outside physician. The airline may also require that passenger medical information be provided on a specific Medical Information Form (MEDIF) for clearance to fly.

GBMS may also be called by the airline to determine if a passenger has a disability that must be accommodated by the airline, or if the passenger has a medical condition that may affect the passenger's ability to safely fly in a commercial aircraft. Recommendations must avoid any discrimination against passengers and ensure the right to free movement [13]. Guidelines for preflight screenings have been published by the International Air Transport Association [14], and specific recommendations regarding preflight medical therapies are provided in Chapter 14 of this book. Individual airlines may also have their own medical guidelines for passenger fitness to fly.

15.3.3 Medical Assessment for Repatriation

GBMS may also be consulted regarding travelers who have developed an injury away from home and need to be repatriated. GBMS may work directly with the insurance company or medical repatriation service to determine if the passenger can travel commercially with or without assistance, or if they require other means of transport such as an air ambulance. This consultation often involves a GBMS physician contacting the treating physician and a collaborative discussion regarding the diagnostic assessment, current treatment delivered, and expected course of care. This information is utilized by the GBMS physician to determine the anticipated medical needs in transport, potential impact of travel such as change in barometric pressure with altitude, and appropriateness of the receiving facility to accept the patient. Separately, the airline may request from GBMS an independent fitness-to-fly evaluation for a passenger that has been booked on that airline for repatriation.

15.3.4 Occupational Health and Crew Fitness for Duty

GBMS has variable involvement regarding occupational health as specified by contracts with individual airlines. GBMS is commonly used to address an immediate crew member's medical issue, as would occur with any other passenger. Other occupational health questions are typically addressed by the medical department of the airline. Alternately, a GBMS center may be contracted to provide a wide range of occupational health services, including determinations of a crew member's fitness for duty. However, only an Aviation Medical Examiner (AME) approved by the Federal Aviation Administration (FAA) may clear a pilot for duty in the United States, whether provided by a GBMS center or directly by the airline.

When a potential medical emergency involves a member of the flight crew, recommendations should always be discussed with the pilot in command to obtain consensus on the best course of action. In some cases, a pilot may be the patient and diversion may be advisable even in circumstances where continuation to destination would be appropriate for a passenger (e.g., syncope) due to concerns over safety of aircraft operations. Medical recommendations provided to flight crew members remaining on duty should take into account that any pharmaceutical treatment must be approved by the FAA as outlined in the FAA Guide for Aviation Medical Examiners [15]. In most cases, the recommendation will be for flight crew members with an ongoing medical concern to be removed from onboard duties, as appropriate considering the type of medical concern, available staff, and needs for safe operation of the aircraft. Upon completion of the flight, airline policies should address the mechanism for a flight crew member to be cleared to return to flight duties.

15.3.5 Public Health Notification

Certain symptom criteria for ill passengers on international and interstate flights may require reporting to a governmental public health agency tasked with protecting the health of the public. In the United States, the Centers for Disease Control and Prevention (CDC) requires reporting of certain conditions to a Regional Quarantine Station on a mandatory or recommended basis (Fig. 15.1) [16]. Similar reporting requirements exist in Canada [17], as well as other countries. These notifications must be made by the airline, though a GBMS provider may assist in recognizing conditions that require reporting and ensure that the appropriate airline staff are notified to make the report.

The GBMS provider cannot override these legal requirements and cannot assume this duty for the airline. GBMS can assist the airline to determine if passenger symptoms meet notification criteria and provide guidance in initial treatment of the ill passenger while in flight. Additional recommendations to cabin crew may be provided to protect against disease transmission, such as use of face masks, gloves, and strict hand hygiene. In some cases, passengers may be moved away from other passengers if space allows.

<u>Required Reporting</u>

- **Fever** (measured temperature above 100°F or 37.8°C) for greater than 48 hours,**OR**
- **Fever** of any duration **plus** any one of the following: rash, swollen glands, jaundice (yellowing of the skin),**OR**
- **Persistent diarrhea**

<u>Requested Reporting</u>

- **Fever** of any duration, **plus**
- **Any one of the following**:
  - persistent cough
  - persistent vomiting
  - difficulty breathing
  - headache with stiff neck
  - decreased level of consciousness
  - unexplained bleeding

Fig. 15.1 Conditions requiring reporting to the CDC when involving international travel to the United States [16]

In the United States, notifications by the airline can be made directly to the CDC Quarantine Station that serves the arrival airport or through the CDC Emergency Operations Center (EOC). The Public Health Agency of Canada has similar regional Quarantine Stations to which their respective reports should be made. Following notification, the public health entity has the authority to quarantine passengers, though this is exceedingly rare. In most cases, information is obtained from the airline, the passenger may be interviewed or evaluated at the airport, and follow-up may be performed as determined by the public health entity.

15.4   Process of Managing an In-Flight Medical Emergency with GBMS

15.4.1 Decision to Contact GBMS

During an in-flight emergency or gate screening, the airline will contact the GBMS center per individual policies and procedures of that airline. Therefore, an event that would trigger a call to the GBMS on one airline may not necessarily trigger a call at a different airline. There are no national or international standards or regulations in place to determine what events warrant contact with GBMS. Also, there is no legal requirement for an airline to contract with a GBMS service in the United States, though most commercial airlines do.

15.4.2 Communications Systems Between Aircraft and GBMS

The flight crew, most commonly the pilot in command, will initiate communication with GBMS via radio, satellite phone, or the Aircraft Communications Addressing and Reporting System (ACARS). Once communications are established, the consultation may be led onboard by the pilot in command, copilot, or other flight crew member. In all cases, the pilot in command remains in contact with all crew members managing the medical emergency and communicates with the GBMS provider regarding all major recommendations.

Radio communications are typically established through regional communications centers. Examples in the United States include Atlanta Radio (Atlanta, GA) and Aeronautical Radio, Incorporated (ARINC, located in New York City and San Francisco). The regional communications center will typically patch the radio frequency onto a telephone line and facilitate a bridged communication with the GBMS center. A consideration in using radio communications is that different frequency bands are utilized for different parts of the United States and Canada, as they are across the world. As the flight moves away from one radio tower, the signal may fade and the aircraft may need to switch frequency. Gaps in ability to communicate may occur.

Satellite phone is a commonly available alternative to radio communications and can provide direct communication between the cockpit, dispatch, and GBMS. Usually it is the most efficient means of communication, yet satellite positioning may limit the ability to communicate and lead to dropped calls. It is not normally used over continental North America, where the radio network is easily accessed by aircraft; instead, it is used more commonly for transoceanic flights.

ACARS provides the ability to send and receive text-based messages between the cockpit and the airline's dispatch center. ACARS may be used when other forms of communication are not available, or to send follow-up information such as age, name, and seat number. As a non-QWERTY keypad is used, ACARS is not ideal for providing lengthy reports. However, when radio and satellite communications are not available or readily accessed, brief or follow-up medical communications may be provided directly to and from the aircraft via the airline's dispatch center by means of ACARS.

Internet communication systems are increasingly becoming available on commercial airlines. While these communications systems are not typically used by the flight crew in the cockpit to establish ground communications, they may serve as an additional mechanism for the cabin crew and medical volunteers to communicate with GBMS.

15.4.3 Management of an In-Flight Medical Emergency Utilizing GBMS

An event begins when a passenger has a medical event and a flight attendant either notices or is informed of the event. The flight attendant must determine if the event requires GBMS notification per the airline's policies. The nature of the event and airline policies also influence whether the flight attendant asks for an onboard medical volunteer to assess the passenger and assist in the management of the medical emergency. Variation exists across the industry regarding the solicitation of medical volunteers; many airlines will routinely request onboard assistance while others will only do so either based upon the type of IME or via guidance from the GBMS.

Upon assessment of the situation, the flight attendant will contact the flight deck and notify the pilot in command. The flight deck contacts the airline dispatch center through one of the previously described communication systems, provides notification of the nature of the event, and requests contact with GBMS. If radio communications are used, the regional radio communications center will simultaneously connect the GBMS center and the airline dispatch center. When using satellite phone communications, airline dispatch is called directly by the aircraft and connects with GBMS.

The GBMS medical provider will obtain information about the medical emergency from the flight crew. This information may be provided from the pilot, from the flight attendant, or directly from a medical volunteer. Additional information may be requested by the GBMS medical provider, as well as an update on the passenger's condition if specific interventions have already been performed or if time has lapsed from initial assessment of the passenger.

Once the GBMS medical provider has enough information, recommendations may be provided regarding general medical care, including use of onboard oxygen and administration of medications from the onboard emergency medical kit. The GBMS provider will be familiar with the location of medications and other equipment within the kit and can facilitate locating the medications, ensure appropriate dosing and route, and identify anticipated treatment effect or potential complications. When recommendations are provided by an onboard medical volunteer, the GBMS provider may be consulted by the flight crew. GBMS may also ensure that the interventions asked of a medical volunteer are appropriate for their level of training, such as starting an intravenous infusion or administering certain medications. Additional recommendations may include whether to divert the aircraft or continue to the intended destination. GBMS can specifically determine the medical capabilities available near airports that are being considered as destinations in a diversion and does this in collaboration with the airline dispatcher. The final recommendation may be to divert to the closest airport, divert to a more appropriate destination based on the patient's condition, or continue to the intended destination if time to the intended destination is not determined to be medically significant for the patient's condition. Finally, GBMS may provide recommendations as to whether emergency medical services (EMS) should be contacted to meet the aircraft at the gate upon arrival. This recommendation may be influenced by the immediate need for additional medical interventions, a determination that the patient will need to be transported to the hospital, or the need to medically screen the passenger prior to making a connection following an onboard medical emergency.

15.5 Medical Decision Making

15.5.1 Role of the GBMS Provider

In cases where GBMS is contacted, nurses or technicians may directly address preflight screenings, questions about medical equipment such as oxygen concentrators, and handle some IMEs based on protocols established by the GBMS medical director. Physicians may be engaged on all or only selected airline consultations. Regardless of the healthcare provider engaged, the GBMS provider renders a recommendation only. For example, the decision to divert an aircraft due to a medical emergency lies solely with the onboard pilot in command and the airline's dispatch center. The pilot in command also makes the final determination of whether a passenger can board an aircraft, in consideration of the safety of that passenger and everyone else on board. Recognizing their medical expertise, when an airline contracts with a GBMS center, the airline usually relies on the recommendation of the GBMS provider as to what course of action to pursue, thus influencing the final decision of the pilot in command.

15.5.2 Role of an Onboard Medical Volunteer

A medical volunteer refers to a healthcare professional who is a passenger on the aircraft and provides volunteer assistance to another ill or injured passenger on the aircraft. It has been suggested that doctors and other healthcare professionals have a duty to act during an IME [18–21] and, in some countries, this duty is mandated by legislation. In the United States, no legal requirement exists requiring intervention by onboard medical volunteer providers.

The role of an onboard versus ground-based physician may be unclear. First, the type of provider who is accepted by the airline may vary from airline to airline; some airlines may require proof of licensure prior to rendering assistance. The medical volunteer should be sober and able to provide a business card or other identification to the flight attendant. When GBMS is engaged by the aircraft, the primary role of a medical volunteer is to gather information, perform a medical assessment, and potentially administer a medication or perform a medical procedure. In most instances when GBMS are available, management of IMEs is a collaborative partnership. The onboard volunteer performs a medical assessment and facilitates key interventions, while the GBMS physician oversees medical care and assists the flight crew in all IME-related decisions. The pilot in command is the primary incident commander and utilizes the information available from all sources when making critical decisions. Of course, the abilities of the onboard medical volunteer and nature of the IME will impact how the partnership develops in individual cases.

With the goal of providing optimal care, it is recommended that medical volunteers ask flight attendants to ensure that communication is established with GBMS regardless of the seriousness of the medical event [1, 22]. This may include input on use or future replenishment of the onboard medical kit, coordination of ongoing medical care upon arrival, and ensuring appropriateness of any major decisions such as aircraft diversion. Contacting GBMS can also assist in preventing avoidable errors, such as incorrect use of an automated external defibrillator or onboard medications [23].

15.5.3 Decision to Divert an Aircraft

The most impactful decision addressed in handling an IME is whether to divert the aircraft to an alternate destination. While both GBMS providers and onboard medical volunteers may influence this decision, the only 2 personnel with licensed operational control over an aircraft in flight are the pilot in command and the airline dispatcher. All medical providers involved in an in-flight event offer advice to these primary decision makers.

Multiple factors must be addressed when considering diversion for an IME. Factors include the medical complaint, stage of flight, and distance remaining. For example, the average aircraft takes 20–30 min to descend and land from cruising altitude. A flight with 30 min or less remaining will not save any time by diverting to an alternate airport. Additionally, different airports will have different nearby medical facilities and the closest airport may not be located near facilities that would best serve the patient. GBMS should have a database of hospitals near each airport where the airline operates to assist the airline in assessing this information. Additional operational considerations include whether specific airports can handle the type of aircraft involved, as well as weather and/or operational considerations. Thus, dispatch must be involved in assessing and making decisions regarding any potential diversion. In making recommendations, GBMS will weigh the severity and time-dependence of the passenger's medical condition, the distance remaining, and the availability of onboard resources (personnel and medications) to make a suitable recommendation. These factors will be different on each flight. In the case of discordance between the recommendation of a GBMS provider and the pilot in command, the GBMS provider should be mindful of providing a recommendation that is in the best interest of the passenger given the situation, yet not argue with the pilot in charge, who may have additional information and experience in these events, as well as the responsibility of ensuring the safety of all passengers onboard.

15.6 Special Circumstances

15.6.1 Inability to Divert an Aircraft

In certain circumstances, immediate landing for medical assistance may be indicated based on the type of IME, yet there may be no suitable place to which to divert the aircraft. This may include flights over the oceans or poles, flights over countries where political or other considerations preclude landing, or situations where it is unsafe to immediately land as is the case with overweight aircraft soon after takeoff. In these cases, GBMS can serve as a resource for continual reassessment and management of the onboard medical emergency through periodic updates from the flight crew. Additionally, GBMS will often work with the airline dispatcher to determine alternate suitable locations for diversion that may become available along the aircraft's route or alter the aircraft's course.

15.6.2 Passenger Death

GBMS may be contacted for a medical event where the passenger shows no signs of life despite efforts by the crew and medical volunteers. GBMS can ensure that appropriate interventions have been performed based on the capabilities of the onboard personnel and the available equipment. If no further care is likely to result in return of circulation, it may be medically appropriate to cease resuscitation efforts. In these cases, neither the GBMS medical provider nor the onboard medical volunteer formally pronounce the patient dead, as they will likely not be present to sign the death certificate, nor have the authority to do so in the jurisdiction where the patient arrives. This process should be undertaken by the appropriate emergency medical service where the flight lands by following local procedures.

If resuscitation efforts have ceased and there are no signs of life, there is no longer a medical reason to divert the aircraft. An automatic diversion may create additional problems, particularly regarding disposition of human remains across national borders. However, there may be other company reasons to divert, including crew exhaustion, biological contamination, or other operational concerns. Diversion decisions in these circumstances should be made by the pilot in command in collaboration with airline dispatch, GBMS, and other airline personnel as warranted. The handling of passenger remains will then be determined by airline policy and local procedures upon flight arrival.

15.6.3 Emergency Medical Kits

FAA regulations require all aircraft with a maximum payload capacity of more than 7,500 pounds and with at least one flight attendant to carry a first-aid kit, an emergency medical kit, and an automated emergency defibrillator (AED) [24]. The FAA has established minimum requirements for the contents of the EMK (Table 1.1). While airlines must maintain the minimum required contents of these kits, they may also add medications and equipment to their individual EMKs. These may include medications for nausea, a glucometer, or a pulse oximetry device. Kits may be individualized for longer or shorter routes. EMKs may be produced by the individual airline or purchased from a third-party vendor.

GBMS centers commonly provide recommendations to airlines they are contracted with regarding additions to their EMK, based on patterns of usage and medical opinion. Airlines make the final decision on the contents of their EMK and must consider the baseline regulatory requirements, as well as the additional cost, weight, and anticipated life span of the medication or device being considered. This must be weighed with the anticipated clinical usefulness and frequency of use. The GBMS center may be able to provide data to inform these decisions.

It is not typically the role of GBMS to prescribe specific medications to individual passengers for the purposes of initial use or replacement. Controlled substances present additional regulatory and security concerns, and some airlines have removed them from the EMK. When the GBMS center also sells EMKs to the airline, the airline should be aware of any potential conflicts of interest. Unnecessary utilization of the EMK contents may increase the cost for the airline. Airlines should have established policies and procedures to determine the location of the EMK, whether it is locked for storage, and who may access the kit during an IME. Most commonly, the lead flight attendant has the key to access the EMK from a locked storage compartment that is usually near the front or rear of the aircraft. Airlines may have policies in place that require contact with GBMS prior to use of the EMK by a medical volunteer or any member of the flight crew, to ensure appropriateness of use and mitigate the risk of providing onboard medical interventions.

Many airlines also may carry a "flight attendant pouch" or "over-the-counter kit." These kits are separate from the EMK and often are stocked with commonly used medications such as acetaminophen, ibuprofen, and antacids. These additional kits allow for the availability of common medications without having to break the seal on the required EMK, thus saving the EMK for a more serious event. The situation of having to send the EMK out for restocking when only a simple over-the-counter medication was needed is also minimized. The availability and contents of these supplemental kits will vary by airline and are not required by the FAA. If utilized by the airline, GBMS should have knowledge of the content of these kits as well.

15.6.4 Emergency Oxygen

FAA regulations also require passenger aircraft with at least 1 flight attendant to carry bottles of oxygen. The actual purpose of this oxygen is to be used by flight attendants in the event of a cabin depressurization to perform their cabin duties. Over time these oxygen bottles have also become thought of as "emergency oxygen" for passengers in need. These bottles come in various sizes and the number of bottles onboard is determined by the size of the aircraft and distance to be traveled. These bottles usually have a fixed regulator to provide low (2 L/min) and high (4 L/min) flow. There is no requirement for an airline to be able to provide continuous oxygen to a passenger for the duration of a flight.

In the event a passenger requires oxygen aboard a long-distance flight, GBMS can assist the flight to calculate the duration of oxygen therapy remaining based on the number and types of bottles available on the aircraft. In rare instances, diversion may be recommended if it is determined that continuous oxygen therapy is required for treatment of the affected passenger and not available in sufficient quantity to last for the remainder of the scheduled flight. In other cases, it may be determined that a passenger in severe respiratory distress cannot be adequately treated with the maximal delivery of oxygen available. GBMS must coordinate with the pilot in command and the airline dispatch to determine if the flight can continue or if diversion is recommended. GBMS may also assist the airline by recommending or coordinating the mobilization of emergency medical personnel on the ground at the receiving airport for continued oxygen therapy based on the passenger's condition.

15.7   Data Collection and Documentation

Limited documentation and reporting of IMEs has been identified as a barrier to improving recommendations for commercial airlines [25, 26]. On an individual case basis, GBMS needs adequate transmission of information from the passenger cabin, which often occurs through relay mechanisms involving the cockpit crew. The sooner and more accurately that information about the medical event can be provided, the sooner a recommendation can be made by GBMS. Without a structured method to obtain and communicate information to ground-based providers, GBMS may be faced with missing information that results in delays to formulating recommendations for the aircraft. Inaccurate information may lead to inappropriate recommendations and potentially result in an unnecessary diversion.

In order to help the process, many airlines have developed a documentation form to capture pertinent data during an IME. Because there are no universal requirements for this documentation, many airlines have developed proprietary forms that are utilized aboard their aircraft (a sample of relevant data elements is provided in Fig. 15.2). The GBMS provider will need to be aware of each client airline form, the data that will be collected, and the expectations of how that information will be transmitted. Airline policy and training should be tailored to maximize the accuracy and completeness of information gathering prior to initiating contact with the GBMS provider.

Data collected on the form may be slid under the cockpit door, where it is communicated to GBMS upon initial contact. When information is complete and comprehensive, GBMS can often make an initial recommendation to the flight without the need for additional information. If the form is not complete and for more complex cases, GBMS may need to request more information. Obtaining this additional information may require a cumbersome relay of questions and information between the cockpit and cabin crew before transmission to the GBMS provider. Airlines should emphasize the importance of accurate and complete information in their initial and recurrent training to ensure that a completed form is provided to the cockpit whenever possible in order to avoid unnecessary delays in the management of these cases. When radio headsets are available for direct communications between the flight attendant and GBMS, airlines should continue to emphasize the use of a standardized data collection form. The signal obtained via a headset in the cabin crew can be of poor quality and incomplete data can again create delays in recommendations for treatment. Furthermore, establishment of a standardized set of data elements that are pertinent to most IMEs can streamline the acquisition and transmission of information regardless of the provider and method of communication between the aircraft and GBMS.

Life threats	Is CPR in progress?
	Has an AED delivered a shock?
Passenger	Age
Demographics	Gender
Medical Problem or	Primary complaint
Symptoms	Associated symptoms
	Duration of symptoms
Vital Signs	Heart rate
	Blood pressure
	Respiratory rate
Medical Volunteer	Presence of a medical volunteer and type?
In-flight Treatment	Oxygen therapy administered?
	AED pads applied?
	Medications administered?
	Other treatment?
Communicable Disease	Presence of Fever (>100.4°F) for 48 hours or longer?
Symptoms	Presence of Fever (>100.4°F) with other symptoms (e.g. rash, vomiting, diarrhea, jaundice, altered mentation)?
Passenger & Flight	Passenger Name
Information	Flight Number
	Seat Number

Fig. 15.2 Sample information contained in an airline medical assistance form

The airline may also work with GBMS to identify key medical conditions that require immediate notifications from the cockpit without obtaining additional information. These may include cases involving:

AED use with shock delivery
CPR on an unresponsive patient
Active labor with imminent delivery of a fetus
Uncontrolled arterial bleeding

These conditions may require immediate intervention and possibly immediate diversion.

In addition to the value of in-flight data collection forms for communication among aircraft crew and with GBMS, these forms are typically stored by the airline as a means of data collection on IMEs. Aggregate data can then be compiled regarding cases encountered by an airline. In addition, GBMS centers will record their own data regarding all consultations by airlines. Aggregate data from these centers have allowed for large descriptive studies on characteristics and outcomes of IMEs [4–8, 27].

Confidentiality of patient information is an important consideration affecting the relationships between GBMS, airlines, and passengers. Information obtained by airline personnel during a passenger screening or IME is utilized by GBMS for medical decision making through contract with the airline. The Health Insurance Portability and Accountability Act of 1996 (HIPAA) does not preclude the sharing of such information with GBMS. There may be a misconception among medical volunteers in-flight or EMS providers on the ground that HIPPA prevents them from sharing patient information; this is incorrect. If the medical provider has a concern about sharing passenger information, the provider can always get permission from the passenger who is seeking medical attention, thus alleviating any concern regarding patient confidentiality.

15.8 Telemedicine and Future Data Transmission with GBMS

As technology continues to advance, there will be opportunities for advancement in the transfer of information to GBMS. As aircraft increasingly incorporate Wi-Fi capabilities, they may have the means to transfer data via a secure Internet method. Several companies currently manufacture devices for telemedicine services aboard aircraft, including transmission of patient medical data, audio, and video from the aircraft. Medical data may include passenger vital signs, glucometer readings, and 12-lead EKG transmissions. These are not yet widely utilized among commercial aircraft.

The theoretical benefits of telemedicine devices must be weighed by the airline against their cost and frequency of utilization. In addition to considerations of improved passenger care, the greatest cost-benefit to the airline would be prevention of diversion. There may be a particular benefit of these devices on long transoceanic flights where diversion is not an option and more advanced medical care may need to be delivered on board as directed by GBMS. However, no data currently exists demonstrating the outcome benefit or cost-effectiveness of these devices. As technology evolves and data is obtained regarding their use, telemedicine devices may increasingly be used aboard commercial aircraft. Other existing technological solutions are also being explored, including the transmission of photographs or digital transmission of the airline's medical event form using the existing Internet network of the aircraft.

15.9 Liability for GBMS Providers

A GBMS provider is contracted and compensated for making a medical recommendation based on the data provided. While medical volunteers aboard domestic flights and flights involving US carriers are covered by the Aviation Medical Assistance Act of 1998 [28], GBMS providers may not be similarly covered. GBMS entities and the physicians involved have been subject to lawsuits following their management of IMEs (Bintz et al v. Continental Airlines) [29],

(Baillie v. MedAire Inc) [30]. Physicians that provide GBMS services should have medical liability coverage as is needed in other patient care settings.

15.10 Quality Assurance and Improvement

Performance of quality assurance and improvement is a key role of GBMS in providing medical advice to airlines. GBMS centers should track and record data on consultations by airlines to continually advise on improvements that airlines can make to best care for ill passengers. There should especially be tracking of aircraft diversions, both because these cases represent the most serious cases for passengers and also the most impactful instances for the airline. It is beneficial for the Medical Director of a GBMS center to receive a daily report of diversions that occurred in the preceding 24 h. Diversions should be reviewed to ensure appropriateness of medical decisions and to provide feedback to the GBMS provider if needed.

While each IME is unique, the GBMS Medical Director should ensure uniformity of care as much as possible among GBMS medical providers. This is particularly important in determining what criteria are used to recommend a diversion and providing consistency in those challenging decisions. The Medical Director also needs to review any cases where a passenger was cleared to fly and then had an in-flight event or diversion. Diversions initiated by the pilot in charge prior to contacting GBMS should also be tracked and reported back to the airline for feedback on flight operations. Finally, tracking the usage of medications and other medical equipment can continually inform recommendations for enhancements in the contents of the EMK.

While assessment of patient outcomes after in-flight medical emergencies is not required or commonly available, airlines may obtain outcome information for quality assurance purposes. The GBMS center may assist in collection of this information for the airline. For example, airlines may routinely obtain information as to whether a diversion occurred on an aircraft following a passenger preflight screening, whether a passenger was transported by EMS following an IME, and if the passenger was admitted to the hospital. Different airlines will have different requirements. Such standardized data collection can facilitate outcome data analysis of IMEs beyond the characterization of IME events [4].

Conclusions

Management of in-flight medical emergencies requires the successful interaction of multiple personnel in a unique environment. Ground-based medical support serves a critical role through contracts with most commercial airlines to provide medical recommendations for the pilot in command, flight crew, and airline dispatch. Even when there are onboard volunteer healthcare providers to directly assist the patient, GBMS can provide expert advice on management of these unique situations. GBMS is commonly utilized by aircraft personnel to make critical decisions, including use of onboard medical equipment and whether to divert the aircraft for immediate medical attention. Contact with GBMS should be considered for management of any in-flight medical emergency.

References

1. Silverman D, Gendreau M. Medical issues associated with commercial flights. Lancet. 2009;373:2067–77.
2. Rayman RB, Zanick D, Korsgard T. Resources for inflight medical care. Aviat Space Environ Med. 2004;75:278–80.
3. Lyznicki JM, Williams MA, Deitchman SD, Howe JP III. Inflight medical emergencies. Aviat Space Environ Med. 2000;71:832–8.
4. Peterson DC, Martin-Gill C, Guyette FX, et al. Outcomes of medical emergencies on commercial airline flights. N Engl J Med. 2013;368:2075–83.
5. Brown AM, Rittenberger JC, Ammon CM, Harrington S, Guyette FX. In-flight automated external defibrillator use and consultation patterns. Prehosp Emerg Care. 2010;14:235–9.
6. Matsumoto K, Goebert D. In-flight psychiatric emergencies. Aviat Space Environ Med. 2001;72:919–23.
7. Rotta AT, Alves PM, Mason KE, et al. Fatalities above 30,000 feet: characterizing pediatric deaths on commercial airline flights worldwide. Pediatr Crit Care Med. 2014;15(8):e360–3.
8. Baltsezak S. Clinic in the air? A retrospective study of medical emergency calls from a major international airline. J Travel Med. 2008;15:391–4.
9. Szmajer M, Rodriguez P, Sauval P, Charetteur MP, Derossi A, Carli P. Medical assistance during commercial airline flights: analysis of 11 years experience of the Paris Emergency Medical Service (SAMU) between 1989 and 1999. Resuscitation. 2001;50:147–51.
10. Gong H Jr, Mark JA, Cowan MN. Preflight medical screenings of patients. Analysis of health and flight characteristics. Chest. 1993;104:788–94.
11. Naeije R. Preflight medical screening of patients. Eur Respir J. 2000;16:197–9.
12. Orford RR. Preflight medical screening of patients. Chest. 1993;104:658–9.
13. Newson-Smith MS. The legal implications of preflight medical screening of civil airline passengers. Aviat Space Environ Med. 1997;68:923–5.
14. IATA Medical manual. International Air Transport Association. 2016. https://www.iata.org/publications/Documents/medical-manual.pdf. Accessed 12 Dec 2016.
15. Federal Aviation Administration. Guide for aviation medical examinters. https://www.faa.gov/about/office_org/headquarters_offices/avs/offices/aam/ame/guide/. Accessed 12 Dec 2016.
16. Regulations to control communicable disease, 42 USC § 264.
17. Quarantine Regulations Act, 2006 (C.R.C., c. 1368).
18. Cheng J, Dowling P. Helping airline passengers. Doctors have duty to public. BMJ. 1999;318:672.
19. Gardelof B. In-flight medical emergencies. American and European viewpoints on the duties of health care personnel. Lakartidningen. 2002;99:3596–9.
20. Bagshaw M. Passenger doctors in civil airliners--obligations, duties and standards of care. Aviat Space Environ Med. 1998;69:810–1.
21. Newson-Smith MS. Passenger doctors in civil airliners--obligations, duties and standards of care. Aviat Space Environ Med. 1997;68:1134–8.
22. Gendreau MA, DeJohn C. Responding to medical events during commercial airline flights. N Engl J Med. 2002;346:1067–73.
23. Katis PG, Dias SM. Potential error in the use of an automated external defibrillator during an in-flight medical emergency. CJEM. 2004;6:45–7.
24. Policy AC121-33B - Emergency Medical Equipment. Federal Aviation Administration. 2006. http://www.faa.gov/regulations_policies/advisory_circulars/index.cfm/go/document.information/documentID/22516. Accessed 13 Dec 2016.
25. Goodwin T. In-flight medical emergencies: an overview. BMJ. 2000;321:1338–41.
26. Mattison ML, Zeidel M. Navigating the Challenges of In-flight Emergencies. JAMA 2011;305(19):2003–4.
27. Moore BR, Ping JM, Claypool DW. Pediatric emergencies on a US-based commercial airline. Pediatr Emerg Care. 2005;21:725–9.
28. Aviation Medical Assistance Act of 1998. Washington, DC: National Archives and Records Administration, Office of the federal Register; 1998.
29. Bintz et al v. Continental Airlines, Inc. et al, 4:13-cv-00566 (S.D. Tex., 2013).
30. Baillie v. MedAire Inc. et al, 2:14-cv-00420 (D. Ariz, 2015).

Use of Commercial Aircraft for Emergency Patient Transport

16

Laurent Verner, Matthew Beardmore, Tobias Gauss, and François-Xavier Duchateau

16.1 Introduction

Evacuating patients aboard scheduled commercial aircraft is both feasible and cost effective; this mode of transfer should be considered when immediate transfer is unnecessary and other means of evacuation is not possible. Compared to specialized fixed-wing air ambulances, commercial aircrafts offer improved flight stability and allow long-haul flights without refueling stops at a minimum of half the cost [1]. Disadvantages include nonflexible schedules, uncertain availability of seats on flights, and restrictions of the International Air Transport Association (IATA) rules that must be within the internal regulations of each airline [2]. Importantly, the repatriation should not impact the flight's schedule nor expose other passengers to hazards, especially any infectious risks [3]. This chapter describes the various arrangements available on commercial airliners in terms of patient installation and additional oxygen administration and provides notice on medical clearance. The use of commercial airliners for the simultaneous transport of multiple patients is also described.

L. Verner, M.D. • F.-X. Duchateau, M.D. (✉)
Allianz Worldwide Partners, Group Medical Direction, Saint Ouen, France
e-mail: francois-xavier.duchateau@allianz.com

M. Beardmore, M.B., Ch.B. (Hons)
Department of Anesthesiology, Peninsula Deanery, Plymouth, UK
e-mail: mdbeardmore@doctors.org.uk

T. Gauss, M.D.
HEMS, East Anglian Air Ambulance, Norwich, UK

© Springer International Publishing AG, part of Springer Nature 2018
J. V. Nable, W. Brady (eds.), *In-Flight Medical Emergencies*,
https://doi.org/10.1007/978-3-319-74234-2_16

16.2 Various Medical Evacuation Services on Commercial Aircrafts

16.2.1 Installation

Basically, there are two means of transporting patients within the aircraft: seated or lying on a stretcher. Seated patients should be stable enough to travel as a standard passenger, including being able to follow safety instructions, such as putting their seats in upright position during takeoff and landing. Such patients follow the same procedures and route through the airport as normal passengers for aircraft embarkation and disembarkation. Where available, business/first-class seats will provide more comfort and space. They should require a minimum of interventions en route as the environment around a standard commercial aircraft seat is extremely restrictive to medical care. For disabled patients and/or to avoid long walks within the airport, a wheelchair service can be requested. There are three types of wheelchair services corresponding to the level of disability: R, S, and C. The "R" type (for "ramp") offers a service to the bottom of the ramp meaning that the patient should be able to climb the ramp if the aircraft has no direct access via an air bridge to the gate. The "S" type (for "step") offers a service to the top of the ramp requiring the patient to walk to their cabin seat from the aircraft door. The "C" type (for "cabin") offers a service direct to the cabin seat (Fig. 16.1). The "S" and "C" types require medical approval by the airline. The "C" type mandates that the patient is accompanied.

Some airlines offer a specific cabin configuration, allowing the lower leg to be in extension: the frontal extra-seat. This configuration is generally used where the entire cabin is economy class or when the business-class seats do not allow sufficient room to extend the leg. The seat back in front of the patient's seat is lowered, making it possible to extend the leg (Fig. 16.2).

Supine patients are transported on a stretcher, which is a metallic structure with a mattress, fixed on the armrests of three-seat rows in economy class. The patient is conventionally positioned facing the rear of the aircraft on the mattress and securely fastened using an aviation-type multiple-point restraint system. A curtain is usually included to allow some privacy and delineate a dedicated space which is more appropriate for medical care (Fig. 16.3). The most advanced systems allow a certain

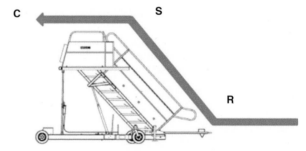

Fig. 16.1 The three types of wheelchair assistance to aircraft seat

Fig. 16.2 Extra seat

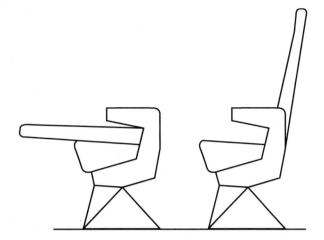

Fig. 16.3 Stretcher

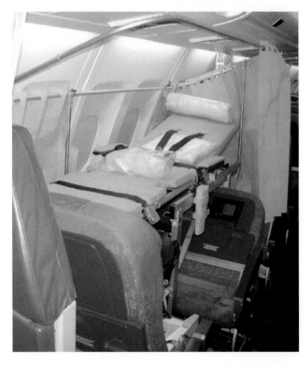

degree of head-up position, though the extent is limited by the distance between the mattress and overhead compartments. The embarkation and disembarkation of the patient use a specific pathway through exit doors at the rear of the cabin to the ambulance on the tarmac. Most airports have a medical lift (Fig. 16.4), but it is important to routinely confirm the presence (and functionality) of such a lift at small airports, since transferring the stretcher is significantly more cumbersome when using a standard ramp.

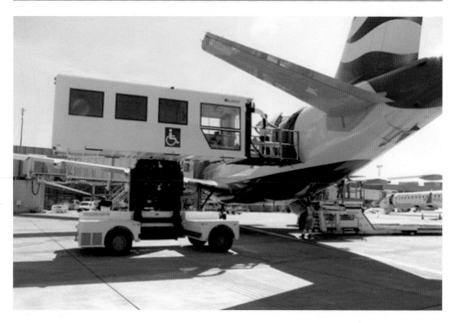

Fig. 16.4 Lift

The Patient Transport Unit is a unique and specific modular system on Lufthansa (within the field of civilian operations) for intensive medical care which requires the removal of seats and installation of bulkheads. This particular unit will not be further detailed in this text since it is much more a specialized air-ambulance module plugged into a commercial aircraft than representative of what is more generally possible on commercial flights.

16.2.2 Oxygen

There are two modes of additional oxygen delivery that can be requested aboard commercial airliners: continuous flow and trigger controlled. Continuous-flow regulators usually offer predefined free flows of 2 and 4 L/min on 2 separate aviation-specific connectors. There are several sizes of tanks, from lightweight handheld portable cylinders up to a maximum of 3,200 L; the latter requires an attachment to the fixing rails on the cabin floor. There is also a specific three-pin quick-release connector to allow the connection of a ventilator. The oxygen-conserving systems provide oxygen for approximately five times longer than the continuous-flow version for the same supply volume. They deliver a pulsed flow of oxygen to the patient triggered by back pressure in the oxygen tubing during exhalation. The efficiency of these devices is of particular interest in the context of long-haul flights and, while they are sensitive enough to function appropriately for most patients, there are situations where the patient will require a continuous-flow regulator.

16.3   Medical Clearance

Unless there is a prior arrangement between the organization providing the transfer and the specific airline, medical approval must be obtained from the medical department of the airline on a case-by-case basis. There is a predefined and IATA-regulated process using standardized forms: Medical Information Form (MEDIF) or INCapacitated passengers handling ADvice (INCAD). These approval forms are to be completed by the treating medical officer or by the medical team responsible for the transfer by delegation. Details regarding the disease, time frames, prognosis for the flight, and special arrangements planned are required. The medical department of the airline approves or declines the transfer request based on this document. This procedure usually takes 24–72 h.

16.4   Use of Commercial Airliners for the Simultaneous Transport of Multiple Patients

In cases of multiple casualty events, the challenge is to quickly set up a large-scale and rapid aeromedical response. Such situations are distressing for both victims and their families, especially when incidents occur in geographical areas with limited medical facilities or capabilities. The response may involve using large civilian jet aircrafts as aeromedical platforms [4, 5].

Although there is a long history of the military transferring large numbers of casualties by fixed-wing aircraft, configuring large civilian jets for aeromedical capability is a relatively new concept. Ideally, aircraft are converted using specifically designed aeromedical modules. There are a few such governmental initiatives [6], but because of the rarity of this situation, many governments or medical providers use makeshift aircraft configurations that can be very effective provided that appropriate coordination and logistical support are applied [7]. One important consideration is the installation of stretchers after the cabin seats have leaned forward, at least in the section of the cabin dedicated to lying patients. This experience showed that the principle of allocating patients to different clinical areas within the cabin is both effective and efficient as it facilitates medical care onboard and streamlines the embarkation and disembarkation procedures [5, 7]. We propose up to three distinct areas: self-caring or minimally-dependent injured patients seated at the front, injured but noncritical patients on stretchers in the middle of the cabin, and the rear of the cabin dedicated to critically ill patients for possible/ongoing intensive medical care.

References

1. Sand M, Bollenbach M, Sand D, Lotz H, Thrandorf C, Cirkel C, et al. Epidemiology of aeromedical evacuation. An analysis of 504 cases. J Travel Med. 2010;17:405–9.
2. IATA. Guidance on managing medical events 2015. https://www.iata.org/whatwedo/safety/Documents/IATA-Guidance-on-Managing-Medical-Events.pdf Accessed 26 Feb 2017.

3. Josseaume J, Verner L, Brady WJ, Duchateau FX. Multidrug-resistant bacteria among patients treated in foreign hospitals: management considerations during medical repatriation. J Travel Med. 2013;20:22–8.
4. Curnin S. Large civilian medical jets: implications for Australian disaster health. Air Med J. 2012;31:284–8.
5. Duchateau FX, Verner L. Response to large civilian air medical jets: implications for Australian disaster health. Air Med J. 2014;33:86.
6. Van Iperen F. Large jet conversions: mass evacuation in the face of changing global medical needs. Waypoint Airmed Rescue Magazine. 2000;13:20–4.
7. Duchateau FX, Verner L. K-plan for patient repatriation after mass casualty events abroad. Air Med J. 2012;31:92–4.

Responding as a Nonphysician Healthcare Provider

17

Edward Meyers, Christin Child, Lisa Bowman, and John Gilday

17.1 Introduction

Your flight has reached its cruising altitude of 35,000 ft, and the drone of the engines is lulling you to sleep. As you are considering the various options to fill your time over the next several hours, you notice activity 2 rows ahead of you. Based upon what you are seeing and overhear, you recognize that a medical emergency is occurring.

As a registered nurse (RN) or as an emergency medical service (EMS) professional (either basic or advanced), your scope of practice and breadth of knowledge are more than ample for most in-flight medical emergencies. With an estimated 44,000 in-flight medical emergencies each year or approximately 1 per every 604 flights [1], being informed prior to departure can help prepare you to better serve your fellow passenger. Are you legally protected in the same manner as your physician colleagues? What can you do to render assistance safely and competently? What tools are at your disposal? Who decides about flight diversion? Given the abundance of questions forthcoming in a scenario such as this, it is important to be aware of the legal aspects of medical care as well as the practical components such as in-flight physiologic changes, what supplies are available, the decision-making process for flight course alteration, and, most importantly, what your scope of practice entails.

E. Meyers, R.N., B.S., M.S.N. EMT-I (✉) • J. Gilday, R.N., M.S.N. NREMT-P
Department of Emergency Services, University of Virginia Medical Center,
Charlottesville, VA, USA
e-mail: ejm@virginia.edu; Jcg6e@virginia.edu

C. Child, R.N., B.S.N., C.E.N. • L. Bowman, R.N., B.S.N., C.E.N.
Emergency Department, University of Virginia Medical Center, Charlottesville, VA, USA
e-mail: CBC3Z@hscmail.mcc.virginia.edu; LMB4S@hscmail.mcc.virginia.edu

© Springer International Publishing AG, part of Springer Nature 2018
J. V. Nable, W. Brady (eds.), *In-Flight Medical Emergencies*,
https://doi.org/10.1007/978-3-319-74234-2_17

17.2 Good Samaritan Laws and the Aviation Medical Assistance Act

Good Samaritan laws do not offer blanket immunity for providers during in-flight emergencies and it is important to note that it is further complicated with air travel given that these laws are state-based and thus may vary. The intent of Good Samaritan laws is to provide immunity to persons who are rendering assistance who are not obligated to do so. However, there are distinct limits to this immunity, and a provider will not be covered when gross negligence or willful misconduct can be proven [2].

Specific to air travel, the Aviation Medical Assistance Act of 1998 (AMAA) was created, in part, to address questions of liability of the air carrier and the passenger rendering medical assistance. While the AMAA focused on such liability, it also identified the need for basic medical training by crew members and the standardization of medical equipment available in flight. In accordance with the AMAA, the airline is protected against liability for the actions of a passenger volunteer so long as the passenger is not an employee of the airline and the flight crew believed, in good faith, the volunteering individual was qualified to render medical assistance. In determining whether a volunteering individual is indeed qualified, it is at the airline's discretion as to whether to allow an individual to render assistance without demonstrating appropriate licensure or certification. Flight attendants may ask for written proof of qualification such as a state-issued license, particularly prior to allowing access to more advanced supplies such as the emergency medical kit (EMK) or the automatic external defibrillator (AED).

As for the passenger volunteer, assuming he or she is licensed or certified, the volunteer is also protected in federal and state courts for acts and omissions unless gross negligence or willful misconduct can be established. Because the AMAA specifically defines "the term 'medically qualified individual' [to include] any person who is licensed, certified, or otherwise qualified to provide medical care in a State, including a physician, nurse, physician assistance, paramedic, and emergency medical technician" [3], this does leave an area of uncertainty related to individuals such as medical students or nursing students. While they may hold a certification such as Basic Life Support, they are not yet considered licensed providers, and the flight crew may find their qualifications insufficient to render care, have access to the supplies onboard, or provide medical recommendations. If given permission to treat the patient, it is the student volunteer's responsibility to recognize their limited qualifications and experience and inform both the crew and patient of such [4]. Should the passenger not consent to treatment, a volunteer can be held liable for battery if they proceed to touch the patient to obtain vital signs or perform a physical exam against the patient's wishes [5]. Ultimately, it is the airline's responsibility for responding to a passenger who has become acutely ill. The role of the medical volunteer is to assist the crew, not to take control of the situation [6].

17.3   Scope of Practice

If responding to an in-flight emergency, a medical volunteer must be aware of and be prepared to act within their scope of practice as defined by the license that they hold. As a nurse or EMS professional, this would include basic lifesaving measures and supportive care congruent with the situation encountered. Depending on the medical emergency, this could include providing orange juice to a passenger with a presumed low blood sugar, placing a patient who has had a syncopal episode in a position of comfort on the floor with legs raised to increase blood flow, providing compressions to a patient without a pulse, or other interventions within a RN's scope of practice. Because of the need for a physician's order for medication administration, one should not give medications provided by the airline unless ordered to do so by a physician. Similarly, as an EMS professional, these stipulations also apply. When responding to an in-flight emergency, a RN or EMS professional may administer care within their scope, but should always be cognizant not to perform any interventions or treatments that they have not been trained to do.

As discussed, the AMAA assures that "an individual shall not be liable for damages in any action brought in a Federal or State court arising out of the acts of omissions of the individual in providing or attempting to provide assistance … unless the individual … is guilty of gross negligence or willful misconduct" [3]. It is crucial to note that this does not offer blanket immunity for an individual knowingly acting outside of their scope. While a medically-qualified individual is defined by the AMAA to include "any person who is licensed, certified, or otherwise qualified to provide medical care in a State" [4], these individuals must still function within their respective scopes of practice in order to be protected by the laws established. Bearing these stipulations in mind, however, it is still possible to provide safe and lifesaving care at 30,000 ft.

17.4   What Can You Do?

Regardless of one's level of practice, the patient and provider relationship begins with an assessment. The scene is first assessed for provider safety and, assuming safety is established, one begins the clinical assessment. The guiding principles of everyday practice still apply; consent, whether it is actual or implied, is required prior to engaging in a patient–provider relationship and, above all, one must do no harm.

Depending on the scenario, an initial assessment is sometimes brief as in a case of cardiopulmonary arrest or potentially more detailed when a case of chest discomfort is encountered. Too often, providers focus on the equipment and medication interventions while glossing over the value of a thorough patient history, a focused physical exam, and a good differential. Providers must also remember that medication administration and many clinical interventions require a physician order in order to remain within one's scope of practice and avoid questions of liability.

Beyond the airplane itself, aircraft have air-to-ground medical communication capability and most have preestablished medical command contracts with a ground physician network to provide orders in-flight as well as to serve as a consult for possible diversion or flight course alteration. As a clinician providing in-flight assistance, it may be necessary to subsequently convey the clinical situation and findings to the ground-based medical services over the radio [7]. Communicating a clear picture will be made easier with a thorough assessment and a detailed clinical history. Once a complete assessment has been conducted, clinical planning, implementation, and reassessment with onboard or remote medical command can begin.

17.5 What Supplies Are Available?

After volunteering to help during an in-flight emergency, the volunteer has a variety of equipment available for use in flight as mandated by the Federal Aviation Administration (FAA) for all passenger-carrying aircraft with a payload capacity exceeding 7,500 pounds and staffed with at least 1 flight attendant. The aircraft is required to have a basic first-aid kit that includes items such as dressings, bandage scissors, and splints. The number of first-aid kits per flight is regulated by the FAA and is dependent on the maximum number of passengers that may be carried on the type of aircraft.

Each flight is also required to carry an EMK which contains medications commonly used in advanced cardiac life support (ACLS), intravenous supplies, a stethoscope and sphygmomanometer, and airway supplies including a bag-valve mask, oropharyngeal airway, and a cardiopulmonary resuscitation mask adapter. In addition to ACLS medications, such as atropine and epinephrine, the EMK also contains oral and IV antihistamines, nitroglycerine tablets, aspirin tablets, a bronchodilator metered-dose inhaler, and dextrose. While these are the regulated requirements, some airlines elect to supply additional medications in their EMK such as ondansetron, glucagon, and naloxone.

In a true in-flight emergency, this kit would contain all the supplies available to the volunteer. Because safe use of the contents requires training beyond the layperson's understanding, these kits are only to be used by medical professionals. Apart from the EMK, an AED is also a required equipment to be on board. However, the AEDs are not required to have a screen displaying the electrocardiogram (ECG), so determining a cardiac rhythm to provide more focused care may not be possible. The EMK and AED are "no-go" items and therefore must be carried on the aircraft as part of the minimum equipment list in order to depart [8].

Some airlines have begun carrying the Tempus IC on their long-haul flights, a telemedicine monitoring device that includes blood pressure monitor, pulse oximetry, thermometer, glucometer, and 12-lead ECG. With recent advances in telemedicine, this device allows for advanced monitoring and communication between the in-flight patient and team and ground crews. However, the Tempus IC is not yet a required equipment on aircraft, though it has the potential to significantly change what in-flight medical care entails [9].

17.6   Environment of Care

Caring for a patient on an aircraft presents the clinician with unique challenges not normally encountered in the typical RN, EMS, or other healthcare professional's workplace. The effects of confined space, changes in altitude, vibration, and noise all can create negative health effects for passengers and alter the way a care provider renders aid.

The limited space onboard an aircraft can make it difficult to treat the passenger when an emergency arises. Depending on care needs, moving a patient to an area that provides more room may be necessary. Flight attendants may use able-bodied passengers to assist in moving the sick passenger to the aisle or the galley area, where more space is available for providing care. In addition, onboard wheelchairs are required for aircraft seating more than 60 passengers and may be requested by in-flight volunteers [10].

In terms of cabin pressure, commercial aircraft must be pressurized to an altitude of no higher than 8,000 ft when operating at the aircraft's maximum altitude [11]. At an altitude of 8,000 ft, the partial pressure of oxygen in the atmosphere decreases from 95 to 60 mmHg, as compared to sea-level. The decrease in the partial pressure of oxygen at altitude results in less oxygen available at the alveolar level. This corresponds with a drop in blood oxygen saturation from 97 to 90% [12]. A healthy adult who lives at or near sea level will most likely not notice the change in altitude, but may respond by increasing their heart rate, cardiac output, respiratory rate, and respiratory volume. Some passengers may experience mild fatigue. However, in a passenger with preexisting cardiopulmonary disease, poor circulation, or decreased cardiac output, their compensatory mechanisms may be insufficient. A small drop in oxygen saturation could cause cardiac ischemia, leading to a medical emergency.

As the cabin altitude increases in the aircraft, the amount of moisture in the atmosphere decreases. Adding to this inverse relationship, cabin air is also recycled with no addition of moisture, further drying the air. During longer flights, this can cause passengers to become dehydrated. This dehydration in an already compromised passenger can further exacerbate underlying medical conditions due to increased heart rate and decreased circulating blood volume.

As the cabin altitude increases, gases expand and some passengers may exhibit signs and symptoms related to this increase. From sea level to 8,000 ft, gas will expand approximately 30%. If a passenger has any trapped gases that are unable to escape, they may suffer pain and discomfort in areas such as the GI tract, ear, sinuses, or teeth. Gastrointestinal effects due to gas expansion during an increase in altitude may include belching, flatulence, and abdominal discomfort. An ear block is a common occurrence during an aircraft's descent, especially for passengers flying with seasonal allergies or upper respiratory infections. Within the middle ear, gases expand during ascent and typically escape through the Eustachian tube. During the decent however, the Eustachian tube is far more resistant to air entering the middle ear, which increases the chance of pain, inflammation, and, in severe cases, bleeding from the pressure difference between the middle ear and the ambient pressure [12].

Lastly, the pressure changes can result in pain in the sinuses, most commonly the frontal sinuses, or teeth when trapped gases expand and cannot be released.

Aside from the changes in the cabin environment caused by the increase in altitude, providing care in a commercial aircraft is further challenged by the effects of the noise and vibration found in this setting. An increase in the ambient noise can hamper a clinician's ability to adequately assess a patient using typical techniques. Auscultation, an important assessment technique, is difficult and sometimes impossible due to the increased noise levels on an aircraft. Additionally, the effects of vibration on a passenger may result in an increase in heart and respiratory rates, making it difficult to differentiate between normal changes and changes due to a passenger's preexisting medical condition.

While the unique environment of a commercial aircraft may limit one's ability to care for a patient using normal assessment tools, these limitations can be overcome if the volunteer uses creative thinking when developing a plan of care for the passenger. Understanding the effects of the changes in altitude on sick or injured passengers, and the inherent differences in the environment in general will help guide the volunteer clinician in providing the best care possible while in-flight.

17.7   Definitive Care Decisions

During an in-flight emergency, the role of the volunteer medical professional is to assist the patient and the flight crew with the presenting medical problem. As the medical professional, the volunteer may have resources at their disposal on board to help in the moment with the situation, but he or she may also be asked to consult with ground-based medical personnel as well. These ground-based medical services can provide real-time support for the medical volunteer, and help coordinate care after landing, including transferring a patient to an appropriate receiving facility, if indicated.

These ground consults play a valuable role in the decision-making process, as choosing to divert the aircraft will rarely be at the volunteer's sole discretion. While the volunteer medical professional, as well as the consult service, can recommend that the plane be lowered to a different altitude to improve the passenger's oxygenation, or that the flight be diverted, decisions will ultimately be made by the captain. The captain has many factors to take into account with making a decision to divert the airline due to a medical emergency, including weather conditions, turbulence, air traffic, approach charts, runway length, landing weight of the aircraft, and proximity to appropriate ground medical facilities. Even under ideal conditions, keep in mind that it can require at least 20 min for the captain and crew to land the aircraft [13].

17.8   Handover of Care/Documentation

Whether during the event itself or after, it is important to document the care provided to the passenger. This can help later if asked to provide information about the care given in flight. In addition, it will also help provide information to the ground-based medical crew during in-flight discussions, as well as report to the emergency medical personnel on the ground after the plane has landed to facilitate appropriate handoff of care. It is also recommended to complete any necessary forms from the airline, especially if any of the contents of the EMK have been used, as these must be tracked by the airline prior to a subsequent flight.

Conclusion

It can be a stressful situation to be called upon to help in an aircraft, away from the hospital or ambulance setting in which you are used to providing care. The unfamiliar environment presents many unique challenges, but remember the basics of your training. Sometimes we look for a more complicated answer instead of focusing on the simplest answer that is before us. In many cases, a good assessment is critical, especially when you are the eyes and ears for the ground medical crew providing orders. Ask questions and listen to the person you are treating to get all the information you can. Remember to practice within your scope, and provide the care that you are trained to do, even if the care you render is as simple as providing reassurance to a scared patient.

References

1. Peterson DC, Martin-Gill C, Guyette FX, Tobias AZ, McCarthy CE, Harrington ST, et al. Outcomes of medical emergencies on commercial airline flights. N Engl J Med. 2013;368(22):2075–83.
2. Lazarin M. Up in the air: responding to medical emergencies at 30,000 feet. 2014. http://blogs.aafp.org/cfr/freshperspectives/entry/up_in_the_air_is. Accessed 6 Dec 2016.
3. Aviation Medical Assistance Act of 1998, H. R. 2843, 105th Cong., 2nd Sess; 1998.
4. Bukowski JH, Richards JR. Commercial airline in-flight emergency: medical student response and review of medicolegal issues. J Emerg Med. 2016;50(1):74–8.
5. Derlet RW, Richards JW. In-flight emergencies at 35,000 feet. The california. J Emerg Med. 2005;6(1):14–8.
6. Gendreau MA, DeJohn C. Responding to medical events during commercial airline flights. N Engl J Med. 2002;346(14):1067–73.
7. Carter J. Emergency at 30,000 feet - what you can do. 2007. https://www.acep.org/Clinical---Practice-Management/Emergency-at-30,000-Feet---What-You-Can-Do/. Accessed 10 Dec 2016.
8. Ballough J. Federal aviation administration advisory circular: emergency medical equipment. 2016. https://www.faa.gov/documentLibrary/media/Advisory_Circular/AC121-33B.pdf. Accessed 10 Dec 2016.
9. Liao M. Handling in-flight medical emergencies. 2010. http://www.jems.com/articles/2010/06/handling-flight-medical-emerge.html. Accessed 10 Dec 2016.
10. Electronic Code of Federal Regulations. 2016. http://www.ecfr.gov/cgi-bin/text-idx?SID=380c896ba2b938a6ecf14403222b53a0&mc=true&node=pt14.4.382&rgn=div5#se14.4.382_165. Accessed 10 Dec 2016.
11. Electronic Code of Federal Regulations. 2016. http://www.ecfr.gov/cgi-bin/text-idx?SID=380c896ba2b938a6ecf14403222b53a0&mc=true&node=pt14.1.23&rgn=div5#se14.1.23_1841. Accessed 10 Dec 2016.
12. Clark DY, Stocking J, Johnson J, editors. Flight and ground transport nursing core curriculum. 2nd ed. Denver: Air & Transport Nurses Association; 2006.
13. Alves P. Management of inflight medical events on commercial airlines. 2016. https://www-uptodate-com.proxy.its.virginia.edu/contents/management-of-inflight-medical-events-on-commercial-airlines?source=search_result&search=Management%20of%20inflight%20medical%20emergencies%20on%20commercial%20airlines&selectedTitle=1~150. Accessed 10 Dec 2016.

Index

Printed by Printforce, the Netherlands